Sportsmen and their Injuries

Sportsmen and their Injuries

Fitness, First-Aid, Treatment and Rehabilitation

W. E. Tucker
CVO, MBE, TD, MA, MB, BCh, FRCS

and

Molly Castle

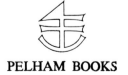

PELHAM BOOKS

First published in Great Britain by Pelham Books Ltd
52 Bedford Square, London WC1B 3EF
1978

ISBN 0 7207 0957 1

Phototypeset in V.I.P. Plantin by
Western Printing Services Ltd, Bristol
Printed in Great Britain by
Hollen Street Press Ltd, Slough, Berkshire

Contents

List of Line Illustrations   7

Forewords   10

Introduction   13

1 On Fitness   15

2 Injuries Common to Most Sports and their First-Aid   34

3 First-Aid in Specific Sports   52

4 The Active Therapeutic Approach to Recovery   92

5 Rehabilitation before Retraining   207

Appendix I: Syndesmology   223

Appendix II: The Skeleton   226

References and Further Reading   227

Index   229

Errata

Page 8   the page reference for Figure 51 should read 165.
Page 9   the page reference for Figures 70 and 71 is 193;
           under 'Figure 77' read 'Dislocation' for 'Discolation'.
Page 74   'Strains and Sprains': line 16 should read 'the outer
           side of the left elbow'.
Page 174   subheading: for 'spondylosis' read 'spondylolisis'.
Page 181   line 19: for 'metatarsal' read 'metacarpal'.
Page 188   line 2: the sentence 'The rest of the movement . . .
           fully pronated.' should be deleted.
Page 227   line 17: for 'De Lorne' read 'DeLorme'.

Line Illustrations

FIGURES
1. Active Alerted Posture   16
2. Inactive Slumping Posture   16
3. Correct alignment of line of gravity forces in Active Alerted Posture   17
4. Alignment of line of gravity forces in Active Alerted Posture is like a well constructed brick wall   17
5. Non-alignment of line of gravity forces in Inactive Slumping Posture   17
6. Non-alignment of line of gravity forces in Inactive Slumping Posture is like a badly built brick wall   17
7. The various positions of the body in perfect Active Alerted Posture   17
8. The six main prime fixing levels of the body with secondary levels at wrist, elbow and shoulder joints   19
9. The spinal column   19
10. Different types of joints   20
11. The weight of the various components of the body   21
12. Right and wrong ways to lift   23
13. Indirect and direct injury to ankle   94
14. The effects of postural strain at the six fixing levels   95
15. Spread of traumatic effusion   96
16. Positive and negative phases of healing in capsulitis of the shoulder   97
17. Manipulation Principle I   109
18. Manipulation Principle II   109
19. Manipulation Principle III   110
20. Manipulation for shortened muscle   110
21. Complications of a large haematoma   120
22. Parallel between the action of a carpenter's plane, smoothing down a thickening, such as a notch, in wood and the 'smoothing', by the Active Therapeutic Approach, of a thickening in the body tissues after injury   123
23. Chronic tenosynovitis, following an acute sprain or direct blow   123
24. Effect of shock strain on alerted and slack muscle   124
25. Neurapraxia   129

26.	Axonotmesis	129
27.	Neurotmesis	129
28.	Effect of direct force at right angles to long axis of bones	130
29.	Indirect violence causing rotatory force producing oblique or spinal fracture	130
30.	Compression fracture	131
31.	Fracture from strong muscular contraction	131
32.	How a stress fracture occurs from a whipping force in the leg bones	132
33.	Positions where stress fractures occur in various sports	133
34.	Fracture reduced and firmly held by a plate and six screws, and an onlay Phemister graft	133
35.	Pearson's Traction	134
36.	Hamilton-Russell Traction	134
37.	Various methods of internal fixation	135
38.	Windows through the plaster of Paris at motor points to enable the administration of surging faradism	138
39.	Plaster for Colles' and Potts' fractures	138
40.	The right ankle and foot from the outer side	141
41.	The tarsal, metatarsal and phalangeal bones (top view)	141
42.	To demonstrate how manipulative and mobilising methods can make a joint such as the ankle one-hundred-per-cent fit in four weeks	144
43.	The right knee (front view)	151
44.	The right knee (inner side view)	151
45.	Genu recurvatum	152
46.	Aspiration of right knee	153
47.	A blow on the outer side of the right knee, causing a direct injury to the outer side and an indirect injury to the inner side	155
48.	Pelegrini-Stieda ossification as a complication of a medial collateral ligament injury	157
49.	How a haematoma will gravitate and cause a synovial effusion	163
50.	How a deep bruising in the muscles associated with the femur can cause periosteal stripping and an organising haematoma resulting in myositis ossificans	164
51.	Front view of pelvis	265
52.	Front view of right hip with right side of pelvis	166
53.	Front view of right hip with ligaments	166
54.	Typical cervical, thoracic and lumbar vertebrae	170

55.	A dorsal vertebra, showing two facets for its rib	171
56.	A fifth lumbar vertebra, showing defect in pars interarticularis associated with spondylolisis	174
57.	A true slip spondylolisthesis	174
58.	How a hairline fracture differs from one with displacement	177
59.	The effects of fracture or bruising of chest wall	179
60.	Front view of left wrist	182
61.	Treatment of fracture of right olecranon caused by strong muscular contraction of triceps: screw fixation placed obliquely	184
62.	Front view of right elbow	185
63.	Right elbow – lateral view	185
64.	Right elbow – ligaments from lateral view	185
65.	Right elbow – medial view	185
66.	To demonstrate how the correctly executed backhand tennis shot is performed by activators acting in conjunction with synergists and prime fixors	186
67.	Right shoulder and right side of chest	192
68.	Ligaments of the right shoulder joint	192
69.	The range of horizontal flexion and extension of the arm	193
70.	Motion of the arm at the shoulder vertical plane showing backward extension and forward flexion	000
71.	Internal and external rotation of the arm	000
72.	The first extension of the shoulder, the inward rotation and adduction	194
73.	Dislocation of right shoulder with head displacing downwards and forwards	196
74.	Manipulation of the shoulder joint	198
75.	Universal sling	198
76.	Fracture of right clavicle treated by screw fixation	202
77.	Discolation of right acromio-clavicular joint	203

Forewords

By John Edrich, MBE, Captain of Surrey County Cricket Club, former Vice-Captain of the England Cricket Team; 102 centuries to date in first-class cricket

It gives me great pleasure to write a short foreword to this book on athletic injuries for my friends Molly and Bill Tucker. Having played cricket for Surrey and England since 1959, I have had my fair share of injuries. As in any sport, one cannot afford to be out of action for very long, so having good treatment is essential.

I have always found that treatment immediately after an injury is very important in establishing sound healing in the shortest possible time. In cases of tears in muscles and strains of joints, I have found that recovery is quick provided full movement and muscle power are restored by physiotherapy and graduated exercises. I have also found that manipulation under an anaesthetic has helped at the appropriate time.

This book tells you how to establish a return to full activity in the shortest possible time.

By Dr R. P. Goulden, specialist in sports medicine

Twenty years ago I had the privilege of joining Mr W. E. Tucker in partnership in his Clinic for Injuries. At first I was very sceptical of his methods, which frequently conflicted with the orthodox conservative methods which I had been taught and previously practised. After six months, however, I realised that the results he achieved, especially in getting the sportsman quickly back into his sport, proved that his theories were sound and surpassed any that I had previously and conventionally used. This is the essence of his approach:

1. The supreme importance of posture.
2. The early disposal of traumatic bruising and oedema so that early

movements can be commenced. This not only prevents adhesions forming but it also allows soft tissues to heal in a fully extended position so that full range of movement can be achieved much sooner.

3. Rest from strain, but at the same time non-weight-bearing exercise without strain to keep muscles in tone until normal weight-bearing can be achieved.

4. Home treatment: encouraging the patient to help his own recovery by removing his splint or support in order to do contrast bathing several times a day. This stimulates the blood supply, and self-massage further helps disperse traumatic bruising and effusion.

5. Graduated remedial exercises under the careful control of a physiotherapist.

The enthusiasm which Mr Tucker manages to instil into his patients to get them to take an active part in their own recovery, his careful supervision and encouragement, contributes much.

By Dr Kevin O' Flanagan, Member of the International Olympic Committee, Executive Member of the International Team Doctors' Association, Chairman of the National Rehabilitation Board of Ireland, Vice-President and Honorary Medical Officer of the Olympic Council of Ireland; capped for Ireland in both Rugby and Association Football in consecutive weeks

I first had the good fortune to meet Bill Tucker when he and I were nominated to serve on the British Medical Committee for the 1948 Olympic Games to be held at Wembley. The year was 1946, and early in 1947 I went to work with him at the London Clinic for Injuries, 21 Grosvenor Square, London W1.

I stayed with him until 1952 when I returned to Ireland to set up my own practice in physical medicine. These years were the most formative years of my life in medicine and to Bill I owe a great deal, not only for his training in Orthopaedic Medicine but for his kindness and friendship which is never failing to everybody he deals with. His generosity is world famous, as is his knowledge in the field of sports injuries in which he is an expert. Most of the well-known sports personalities of the world have at some time or other had cause to be grateful to Bill.

I deem it therefore a great honour to write a few words of the foreword to this book, so ably put together by Bill and his charming wife, Molly

Castle – who is, of course, an acknowledged expert in her field of nutrition, and as an editor.

This book covers everything from minor to serious injuries in every sport, with special emphasis on the value of fitness, early diagnosis, assessment, first-aid, and the initiation of early treatment and eventual rehabilitation and retraining.

The value of home treatment in rehabilitation is of paramount importance and again special emphasis is placed on it. It is amazing how much benefit the injured athlete can gain from it.

We are all very keen on the importance of Active Alerted Posture, particularly for the young athlete, and I think it is especially apt that such tremendous importance has been placed on this chapter. I am still amazed to see top-class athletes who break down with foot trouble as a result of a tendency to stand flat and even to run valgus . . . points which the book continually emphasises.

Molly has made a significant contribution to this book, not only in the chapters on fitness, nutrition and home treatment but also in 'translating' some of Bill's technical terminology into language which the sportsman himself can understand.

It is, however, a book not only for the sportsman but also for the para-medical personnel engaged in all sports and I feel sure it will make a big impact in the sports world and will be avidly sought and read by everyone, including doctors and surgeons concerned with the sports scene.

By the late Dr Austin T. Moore, famous American orthopaedic surgeon, well known in the United States during his lifetime for his knowledge of sports injuries and nutrition

Molly Castle, a former health editor on the *New York Times* Sunday supplement and on *McCall's Magazine*, has spent many years studying nutrition, psychology and posture and she is particularly an authority on nutrition and on other methods of health preservation. She and her distinguished surgeon-husband have personalities that radiate warmth and vitality. They are living examples of the benefits that accrue from practising their way of life.

Introduction
by W. E. TUCKER

When I was first asked to write this book on the prevention of sports injuries and their first-aid, complications and treatment, and the rehabilitation of patients after injury, in a manner that would be easily understood by athletes with little or no medical knowledge, I felt that this would not be easy. My previous books have all been couched in highly technical language and directed to the medical profession. However, my wife, Molly Castle, is an author and journalist who writes on health for the general public and has many times 'translated' my medical jargon. A book written by both of us together should, therefore, be both comprehensive medically and understandable to any sportsman, whether he be a player, coach, trainee, school games master, referee, umpire or in any other way connected with physical medicine and sport. When we use the first person plural it simply refers to the two of us. Women's libbers must not mind if we use 'him' instead of 'her'. This is not discrimination. We are referring to Man, the human species, not man the male object.

We start with fitness in all its phases because we believe that this is the best preventive against injury. We will show clearly the easily recognisable signs and symptoms which indicate that a sportsman should stop being active and come out of the arena; how he should be treated when first injured, even before he has been seen by a doctor; how he can help the doctor in his efforts to rehabilitate him, when it is safe for him to return to his sport. We also devote one large section, chiefly for reference by the medical profession, to a comprehensive survey of the latest techniques in the treatment of sports injuries. We deal further with prevention: guarding against the occurrence of injury; and the prevention of complications after injury which inevitably can sometimes come about if steps are not taken to avoid them. There are certain rules of treatment: although there are many short-cuts to recovery, the basic principles must never be broken.

In the book we cover most of the better known sports, and we recommend that a copy be kept in the first-aid kit of anyone responsible for any group of sportsmen. There are times when an athlete can be too brave, when he will get back into the game, or on his horse, or whatever, because he feels that the show must go on or that he must not let down the side. The person in charge can immediately find in this book authority for ordering the sportsman off the field if any permanent damage might result in his being too stiff-upper-lipped – as well as the reassurance of knowing when it would do him no harm to receive the applause of the returning hero.

Many people will turn first to the section concerning their own sport and only later to the general prevention of injury, the recognition of treatment in a generalised way, and the warning of possible after-effects. Our advice is *don't*. Read the book through, first of all, to get a picture of sports injuries in all their aspects and then later return to your individual sport.

We have received help from many sources and we should like particularly to thank the American Academy of Orthopaedic Surgeons for allowing us to refer to their books *Joint Motion: of Measuring and Recording* and *Emergency Care and Transportation of the Sick and Injured*. We are also grateful to Churchill Livingstone for allowing us to use many of the diagrams appearing in my books *Active Alerted Posture* and *Home Treatment and Posture*. Other drawings were supplied by Mrs Gillian Oliver, to whom we should like to express our thanks.

The following orthopaedic surgeons have been most helpful: Arthur Bernhang, Arthur Helfet, Basil Helal and Ian Smillie; doctors Kevin O'Flanagan of the Irish Olympics Committee, J. L. Blonstein of the Amateur International Boxing Association and R. P. Goulden. We should also like to thank Col. Rudyard Russell of the British Olympic Boxing Committee and Harry Cox, deep-sea diver of Bermuda, and many others who have given us help, suggestions and criticism.

At the end of the book is a bibliography to which readers may refer with benefit if they wish to extend their knowledge.

1
On Fitness

Fitness and Health

Fitness and health are not necessarily the same thing. A person can be perfectly healthy without being able to run a mile in under four and a half minutes, play five sets of tournament tennis or survive an afternoon's football.

Fitness for an athlete is very specific. It implies training, though it can and does include health: no sportsman can train effectively for his sport if he is not completely sound. It incorporates postural training, the elementary knowledge of body mechanics, sound nutrition, general training, preparation for solo sports, group practice for team sports, readiness for special events and the retraining needed after an injury before the sportsman should be allowed to return to full activity.

Postural Training

Sportsmen are possibly aware that correct posture is necessary for co-ordinated movement but very few, except perhaps a gymnast, a tightrope walker or a ballet dancer, realise how essential to their athletic prowess it is to maintain a balanced upright posture. Good posture can also do a great deal to help avoid accidents. Poor, slumping posture contributes not only to indifferent performance but also to the possibility of injury.

There are two kinds of upright posture: Active Alerted, which some adopt naturally but most have to be taught, and Inactive Slumping, which is the stance of most people. That these postures are connected with mind and mood is obvious when you think of a depressed person, eyes cast down, shoulders hunched, and compare him with someone whose mood is

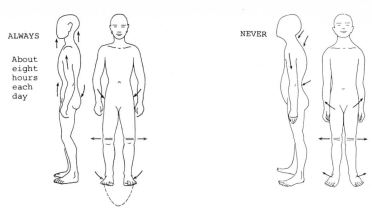

Left: Figure 1. Active Alerted Posture is also balanced, concentric posture. Muscles on opposite sides of the body are in slight isometric contraction. *Right:* Figure 2. Inactive Slumping Posture is also unbalanced, eccentric posture. Gravity strains are not prevented.

confident, who swings along, head up, shoulders back, moving with grace and control. Active Alerted Posture, which is an attitude not only of the body but of the mind, is a complete way of living and moving, promoting both mental and physical equilibrium and poise.

Since man stood upright instead of on all fours, he has had to contend with a greater force of gravity pulling at his joints and internal organs. Gravity is, of course, necessary. Without its force we would be floating around in space like balloons filled with gas. The straighter the line of gravity, and with a reasonable width of base, the more stable we are. As soon as the line of gravity passes outside the area enclosed by the supporting base – for instance if you stand on one foot – the line of gravity will waver outside the base and it is easy to lose your balance.

In order to visualise how the pull of gravity can affect your body, think of a child's tower made of varying sized bricks. If the bricks are placed securely one above the other so that the line of gravity passes through the centre of each of them, the tower can be made quite tall without tumbling; if, however, each brick juts out to one side or the other, or goes too far over in one direction like the Tower of Pisa, it will soon collapse.

One of the great benefits of Active Alerted Posture is that it aligns the 'bricks' one above the other so that the line of gravity is centralised above a firm base. This lessens, to a considerable extent, gravity's downward tug on various parts of the body, such as internal organs and joints. For this reason, it is a posture which makes immediate dynamic action possible. It

16

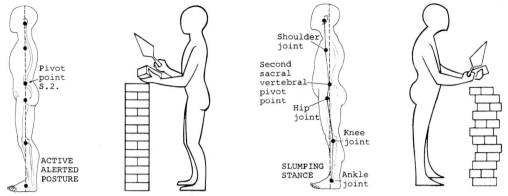

Left to Right: Figure 3. Correct alignment of line of gravity forces in Active Alerted Posture; Figure 4. Alignment of line gravity forces in Active Alerted Posture is like a well constructed brick wall; Figure 5. Non-alignment of line of gravity forces in Inactive Slumping Posture; Figure 6. Non-alignment of line of gravity forces in Inactive Slumping Posture is like a badly built brick wall.

helps to avert accidents due to slow co-ordination of mind and body action.

This is how it is achieved. You stand with the weight evenly distributed on the heels, the outer side of the feet, gripping the ground with the toes. The knees are slightly flexed and act as shock absorbers. The buttocks are tucked under, the pelvis tilted so that it is at right angles to the ground. The shoulders are lifted and relaxed, shrugged slightly forward. The head is held so that the contraction of one group of muscles at the back of

Figure 7. The various positions of the body in perfect Active Alerted Posture.

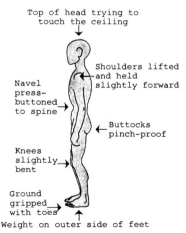

the neck balances the ones in front (isometrically). The chin is tucked in and the back of the neck held straight and lifted so that the top of the head is as if tied to the ceiling.

By making the feet a firm base you will lessen the chance of foot troubles, such as fallen arches, both longitudinal and transverse. You will be able to activate with a spring. In addition, your internal organs will be well supported in the pelvic basin by the balanced contraction of the abdominal, back and buttock muscles.

This posture encourages the full expansion of the lungs by ensuring balanced action between the muscles of the abdominal wall and the diaphragm. The whole process is like a bellows. This means that all the waste products from the bottom as well as the top of the lungs are removed regularly.

The flexible, lifted shoulders will neutralise gravity's pull on the upper limbs, the shoulder girdle and neck muscles. The blood flows more freely to the brain, carrying the oxygen needed to counteract fatigue, poor memory and headaches.

The ability of the body to perform many and complex patterns of motion makes possible the great variety of movements demanded of a sportsman and it is the brain which commands these movements. An ape, for instance, the animal nearest to man, has the physical capacity to perform certain inherited skills and it might possibly be taught to use these to play golf, for example. But it would never achieve the brain power to win an Open Championship.

Fitness and the Mechanics of Movement

It may be easier to acquire Active Alerted Posture if you understand, to a certain extent, the mechanisms of body movement and how these can be used to achieve or enhance certain skills.

The skeletal framework – bones – gives the requisite rigidity to enable the body to resist gravity and maintain an upright stance. Six levels comprise the skeleton: the head on the spinal column; the arms on the shoulder girdle, attached to the neck and trunk; the spinal column on the pelvis; the pelvis on the hips; the top of the body on the knees; the whole body on the ankles and feet. These are the levels where the most strain

18

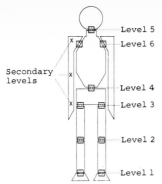

Figure 8. The six main prime fixing levels of the body with secondary levels at wrist, elbow and shoulder joints. These can be called bases, platforms or pivot points.

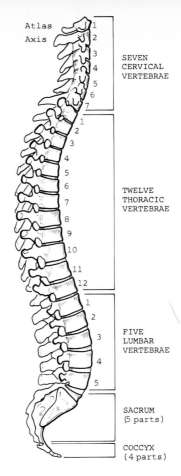

Figure 9. The spinal column.

occurs in the upright position.

The central and perhaps most important of these bony elements is the spinal column, which consists of twenty-four movable vertebrae, five immovable vertebrae fused into the sacrum, and four into the coccyx. Between each two movable vertebrae is a cartilaginous disc starting between the second and third cervical vertebrae and finishing at the bottom lumbar vertebra (the fifth) and the first sacral vertebra.

Bones are covered with a fibrous membrane called the periosteum by means of which muscles and tendons and blood vessels are attached to them. These bones are fastened to each other at the joints: without them the skeleton would be stiff.

There are a number of different types of joint, and the degree of movement possible is dependent on the type. Some joints, in fact, are fixed; some have limited movement; while others, like the ball-and-socket

19

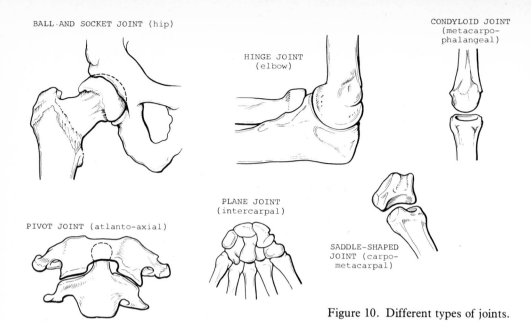

BALL·AND SOCKET JOINT (hip)

CONDYLOID JOINT
(metacarpo-
phalangeal)

HINGE JOINT
(elbow)

PIVOT JOINT (atlanto-axial)

PLANE JOINT
(intercarpal)

SADDLE-SHAPED
JOINT (carpo-
metacarpal)

Figure 10. Different types of joints.

joints of the shoulder and hip, have considerable freedom of motion in all
directions. (See the section on syndesmology, page 223.) Capsules strengthened by ligaments bind the bones together forming the individual joints
so that dislocation is rare. These ligaments combine with the contour of
the bones as well as the overlying muscles and are an important limiting
factor in joint movements. The joints are kept firm and flexible by the
muscles, which are elastic.

Although there are other types of muscles in the walls of the blood
vessels and the alimentary canal, as well as the pumping muscles of the
heart, those of interest in regard to posture are the skeletal muscles,
without which the bones and joints cannot move. You have probably seen,
in medical books, pictures of a person peeled of his skin so you can
visualise the way the muscles are arranged in groups according to their
action. Each muscle consists of millions of fibres woven on to the outside
of the skeleton.

Muscle tissue needs a more rapid turnover of food material than any
other part of the body; the arteries bring the material to the blood stream.
The waste products left over from the combustion of foodstuffs must also
be removed, and this is accomplished by the venous and lymphatic
circulations. As well as the arterial, venous and lymphatic circulations,
fifty per cent of body fluid consists of the fluid within the cells which make

20

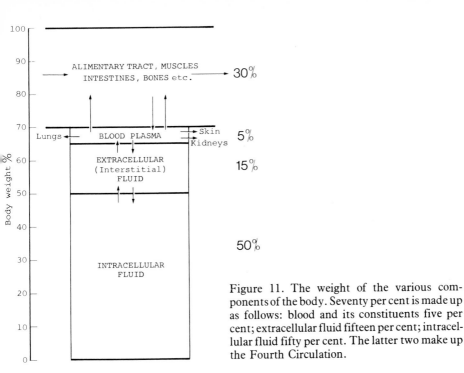

Figure 11. The weight of the various components of the body. Seventy per cent is made up as follows: blood and its constituents five per cent; extracellular fluid fifteen per cent; intracellular fluid fifty per cent. The latter two make up the Fourth Circulation.

up the various tissues. Fifteen per cent is in the spaces between them. We call the two latter ones the fourth circulation.

This circulation is propelled by the pumping action of the skeletal muscles. If, through injury, or inactivity caused by lengthy bed rest, the fourth circulation is diminished and there is the possibility of oedema – the accumulation of excess fluids and metabolites (waste products), in the tissues. The latter tend to cause tissue tenderness, feelings of fatigue and even pain.

A similar condition results following strenuous exercise when the removal of waste products has lagged behind their rapid production, or it may be due to slumping posture when the anti-gravity muscles become fatigued through working at a mechanical disadvantage.

The muscle group primarily concerned with producing any particular movement is called the prime mover or activator. These muscles are

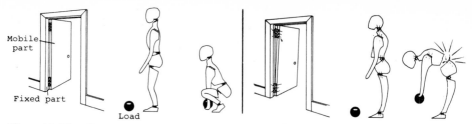

Figure 12. The effects on the body of (left) correct and (right) incorrect ways of lifting may be compared to a door which is mechanically sound (left) and one which is unstable (right). Incorrect lifting may result in an unstable lumbo-sacral level.

assisted by muscles called synergists, but both sets must work on a firm base held steady by the muscles called the prime fixors, as when hitting a tennis ball and kicking a football. For example, if a door were opened before it was firmly attached to the door frame by hinges and screws it would fall away from the frame.

The muscles which restrain or control the given action are called the antagonists. For example, when one group of muscles pulls the forearm upward – flexion – another set of muscles is available to pull it downward again. When you get a contraction of the activating group, the opposite group elongates.

Every movement of which the body is capable is effected by means of this balanced system of opposing muscle groups. When the muscles are in harmony and synchronise perfectly, the movements will be graceful and smooth. Imperfect synchronisation produces awkward, jerky movements. In order to achieve harmony, all muscles must be able to contract strongly and quickly and to relax and lengthen just as quickly.

Muscle tissue is also supplied with nerves: sensory nerves for sensation and motor nerves for movement. Impulses transmitted to the muscle along the motor nerve from the brain cause it to move.

Our bodies have a system of message delivery far more complicated than a telephone switchboard. The part of the brain which is the switchboard or control tower receives messages from all the body senses, co-ordinates the information and then orders changes of position where and when desirable.

Where the body is trained to react correctly – as, for instance, in that of an Olympic sportsman – its movements are co-ordinated at a high level of integration. The control tower in the brain is constantly monitoring and relaying information from various sensory sources and the result may be

22

perfect motion. But even in a less-than-perfect action – a movement, say, performed by a cricketer on the village green rather than one in a Test match at Lord's – a system of action, interaction and reaction almost impossible to visualise is involved.

The movements of an athlete, even of the village-green variety, are seldom simple. They twist and curve and, even in running or walking, flexion and extension of the hip joint are combined with some degree of rotation. Similar mechanisms are at work in the joints of the feet, knees, spine and arms. The athlete, pole-vaulting, running or jumping, has not time to think of all the component parts of a perfect movement; his years of training have made these almost automatic. Almost but not quite. When things go wrong – when Jacklin goes off his game or Billie Jean King is beaten by an unseeded newcomer – someone has to know enough to recognise the cause of it and put it right. This is why their coach or trainer has to have a working knowledge of the mechanics of joint movement so that he is able to spot where things have gone wrong.

There was the case of a famous bowler at cricket who had experienced recurrent attacks of pain in the under surface of his left foot. The pain disappeared in the winter when he was not playing but returned each year as soon as spring practice began. It became progressively worse during the season and was diagnosed as a strain of the spring ligament and the short muscles of the longitudinal arch caused by planting his left foot flat on the ground as he finished the action of bowling – he was a right-hander – so that the foot and the ankle were twisted outward. He was shown how to correct his ankle and foot posture. As he was taking the final step with the left foot he was told to plant the foot firmly on the ground with his weight on the outer side, and at the same time to grip with his toes and turn his foot slightly inward. This had the effect of fixing the foot firmly on the ground so that there was no twisting to strain the ligaments and tendons. Not only did he have no more pain but his bowling improved. It took him a little time to learn the new pattern of distributing his weight on the correct weight-bearing part of his foot, so that his right arm and body had a firm platform from which to work, but once he learned to activate on a firm base he had no more trouble.

A baseball pitcher, who is over-ambitious and under-trained, can suffer from a strain of the muscles on the inner side of the elbow with swelling and pain or, in Little League pitchers, possibly inflammation of the growing part of the humerus bone at the elbow (the so-called 'funny bone'). If he continues pitching incorrectly this may result in serious irrevocable damage to the still undeveloped bone.

In both cases it is the expert trainer who spots the faulty mechanisms in his trainee and shows him how to put these right, or, if symptoms of pain and swelling appear, stops him pitching at once.

The Avoidance and Prevention of Injury

Some injuries are impossible to avoid, of course, and the injured person cannot be held responsible. If a player gets a direct hit from a hard ball he is accountable only if he saw it coming and made an unsuccessful attempt to avoid it.

Some injuries can be circumvented by the use of special skill. If a horse slips, refuses or bucks, he may throw the rider out of the saddle, but a skilful enough horseman can often retain his seat or, at the worst, know how to fall so that his injury is minimised.

Other injuries are inherent in the sport itself. A football player – any type – cannot evade physical contact which could, and often does, damage him. In American football the players, by wearing protective clothing, do a good deal to lessen contact injuries. On the other hand, part of the protective apparel can actually be used as a weapon, especially the helmet which – in some cases illegally – can butt an opponent in the stomach or other parts of the body very painfully. In soccer a collision of two players jumping to head the ball can result in an injury to foreheads, eyes, noses, or in a pulled hamstring, calf, groin or back muscle. It is apparently unavoidable and is much more likely to occur in players who either are not warmed up, not fully fit, fatigued, or are using incorrect posture.

If a perfect action is analysed it is found to be executed in two distinct and separate phases. The muscles which fix the action must be alerted and then the muscles which activate the action (the activators) assisted by their companion muscles (the synergists) can perform on a firm base, without risk of injury to either set of muscles or joints. A good simile is a gun which must be loaded and then, with the safety cock off, can be fired instantly.

If the action is performed before this fixing takes place, there is a danger of muscle strain and strains on joints and eventually perhaps stress fracture. An example of an accidental, unfixed movement is coming down steps in the dark and missing the last step, jarring the whole system.

24

Other accident-provoking afflictions, such as muscle cramps, stitch, foot blisters, sun or heat stroke, can usually be avoided with simple methods.

Muscle cramps in the legs during play may be due to dehydration carrying salt out of the system. Tennis tournament players can often be seen taking salt pills during the crossover. Tight garters obstructing circulation may also be the cause of muscle cramps which are relieved by removing the constricting garter.

A stitch is usually caused by eating too large a meal immediately before taking part in an athletic event. The cure for this is obvious: no large meal for two hours before the event.

Suitable clothing is essential both in hot and cold weather. Covering the head in strong sunlight may avert trouble. Covering the whole body with a track suit or other suitable garments is important in cold weather and may make all the difference to efficiency of performance.

Many pulled muscles are caused by activating in cold weather before the body is warmed up and the athlete should keep his track suit on until his body is really well warmed. Even in the summer, tournament tennis players wear a sleeveless sweater until they are thoroughly warmed up.

Jim Peters, once holder of the world's best marathon time, had a way of preventing tendon trouble not only for marathon and road running but also for distance running. He cut the inner sorbosole out of an old pair of plimsolls and put them into the ones he was wearing. By absorbing the shock, this took much of the strain off the tendons.

To avoid personal injury, the sportsman himself should be as fit as possible before the start of the game or event, learn to fix his movements on a firm base, obey the rules of the sport and hope that others will do the same. An umpire or referee can help here by penalising a dangerous act but he may not be able to prevent it happening in the first place.

Nutrition

Nobody is going to excel in sport unless his body is in good repair. He should have neither too much weight nor too little. The body should also respond instantly and accurately to all commands of the brain. For this, good posture is important; but the right amount of the right foods is equally important.

All foods are used for heating, energy, repair of existing tissues and the creation of new ones where necessary. An athlete's daily intake is often upwards of 4,000 to 5,000 calories – about thirty or forty per cent of which is efficiently used. If this seems a small proportion, it is still four times as efficient as the average motor car. A certain amount is stored, as fat, against a hungry day. Our early ancestors in caveman days had no corner shop and had to depend on their luck out hunting.

During exercise, more heat than usual is provided by the body. It is not exercise itself that warms the body but the waste heat which results from the system providing a little more of everything than is actually needed. When, in those primitive times, fear made the heart, lungs and sweat glands work overtime it was to provide the instant means of 'flight or fight'. This was accomplished by releasing adrenalin into the blood stream. The mechanism still exists today and can be useful in providing an athlete with that extra spark which he needs to win an important event.

There are three categories of food. *Proteins* are needed to build and repair; *fats and oils* for lubricating and for the production of heat and energy; and *carbohydrates* which are also used for energy but can be converted and stored as fat if not used up in activity. The protein group is the most important of the food categories. With almost any reasonably balanced diet the body can borrow a sparking-plug from some other food. What it can't do is to manufacture some of the vital ingredients of protein; these must be provided from outside sources. The biochemists know there are twenty-three essential factors, known as amino acids, which can be strung together in a wide variety of combinations and permutations to form proteins. There is a certain element in protein, however, which cannot be produced synthetically in the test tube. Some nutritionists have even called this the germ of life. This is why, they say, protein foods are of first importance and why, in the under-developed countries, people die because they cannot get enough protein.

At one time it was thought that all athletes required their essential protein in the form of vast quantities of meat. But protein can just as well be obtained from dairy produce – eggs, milk, cheese – and from many vegetable materials – nuts, legumes, root vegetables, and from whole grains. The best protein of all may well be fish, for the Japanese and Hawaiians and other big fish-eating nations can produce just as great athletes as the meat-eating countries. Athletes should eat three servings a day of protein food but are advised not to rely on meat as the sole source.

26

As well as 'oiling the works' fats and oils provide some of the body's energy, from a protective layer round the nerves (which is one reason why a slimming diet containing no fat causes irritability) and act as a medium for carrying the fat-soluble Vitamins A, D and E round the body. Some fats and oils, preferably vegetable and also preferably unsaturated, should be eaten every day.

Vitamin A is needed for eyesight, healthy skin; Vitamin D for strong bones. Vitamin E, for which nutritionists are continually discovering new important uses, has long been known as necessary for the heart and circulation.

Foods containing Vitamin A are plentiful. It comes in leafy vegetables, in the yellow vegetables in the form of carotene which the body changes into Vitamin A. It is also found in butter, margarine, cream, whole milk, eggs and liver (fish or meat). Vitamin D comes from sunshine, fish livers or irradiated vegetable oils. Vitamin E is obtainable from whole grains, wheat germ and wheat germ oil and pressed vegetable oils, especially soya, peanut or sunflower (good for salad dressings).

Carbohydrates are chiefly sugars and starches. Sugar in fruits, milk and honey is better for you than white sugar which has been depleted, in processing, of its vitamins and minerals. Starches are mostly derived from flour. Whole grains: whole wheat, steel-cut oats, brown rice and whole rye are the best ways to eat carbohydrates (starch) because they have not had the goodness taken out of them. White bread is, of course, 'enriched' by the addition of some of the vitamins and minerals that were removed from it. 'Enriched' is rather a misleading word. Anyone who has had £25 stolen from him and £5 replaced may feel grateful for small mercies but is hardly likely to feel enriched.

In their natural state foods are put together in a very clever fashion so that each food is complete with everything in it that the body needs to metabolise it. Man has been very unwise in disturbing the pattern by splitting the foods up, often taking out the very factor without which the remainder is almost valueless. It is as if the sparking-plug of a motor car was removed and the petrol expected to burn anyway.

The chief group of vitamins removed from white flour is the B complex. A great deal is known about this group of twenty or more integrated vitamins and it is said that if the knowledge were universally applied, the improvement in world health would be beyond imagination. Among the group, all of which are found in liver and yeast as well as in whole grains, is an anti-fatigue, anti-stress, anti-anaemia factor and many others which are useful to sportsmen.

Fresh fruit, a useful source of natural sugar (fructose) is also the best source of Vitamin C. One of this vitamin's many functions is to maintain collagen, a strong, cement-like material which binds every cell in the body. Strong connective tissues are important to the athlete who probably receives more minor injuries than the unathletic type. The ability to mend broken bones is helped by Vitamin C. One well-known American orthopaedic surgeon, whose practice was largely among footballers and water skiers, advocated a 'cocktail' of citrus fruit, eggs and powdered milk (for calcium) whenever he had to treat broken bones.

An excellent carbohydrate food is the Swiss cereal muesli (there are many varieties on the market), which is made from several whole grains – wheat, rye, oats – various nuts, honey or Barbados sugar and dried fruits, and which is especially valuable nutritionally when eaten with cottage cheese, live yogurt and/or whole milk.

A balanced diet consists of a wide selection from each of these categories daily. From the protein group at least three servings of meat, fish or eggs; two from the dairy – milk or cheese. From the fat section, margarine or butter, salad oil, fish oil. From the carbohydrate category, whole grains, fresh fruit and vegetables (cooked and raw) in abundance. An athlete using, in energy, upwards of 4,000 to 5,000 calories a day is not likely to go short of vitamins on a balanced eating plan. Nor should he need anabolic steroids: these were once advocated to strengthen muscle power and favoured by weight lifters, among others, until their use was stopped as part of the movement against artificial drugs.

The human body is very flexible and can break down any food into its essential ingredients for growth, maintenance and repair, but it needs a selection from which to choose everything it needs. If the components are not adequate – if 'straw' is provided instead of 'bricks' – the repair work will still be done but it will not be as lasting or as satisfactory.

Yet different peoples survive on very different selections, from blubber, to rice, to fruit and nuts – as long as they get some protein they can live, if not always healthily. Healthy, adequate diets can vary widely also. The Japanese like raw fish and rice, the Italians spaghetti and veal, the British meat and two veg. and plenty of bread. As a result of air travel and occupying armies, however (as has happened in Japan), diets have become more standardised on a world-wide basis, though this is not always to the best advantage. There is still, however, a certain problem for the catering departments during international sports gatherings. In fact the caterers have more of a problem than the human body with its infinitely complicated engineering process of conversion.

General Training

For almost all sports a period of general training at the beginning of the season, after a rest period, is necessary. The athlete has to work at raising the level of his achievement to within sight of his ultimate goal. Unless he has been sensible enough to cut down on his intake of food during the rest period, when his output of energy was lessened, he may be overweight. The only efficient way to reduce is to cut down on the amount of food and step up the output of energy by exercise.

Most doctors and coaches advise a period of graduated exercise to work up to full activity. Weight lifting, walking, jogging, interval running (Swedish *fartlek* or 'speed play') can all be part of a useful programme at the start of training. In addition, most people interested in their own fitness do a daily dozen and there are a great many systems which exercise muscles not usually reached in everyday living: Isometrics, Mensendieck, Yoga, the Alexander Method, the Canadian Air Force Method, and others. Most people have their favourite routine. Breathing exercises are also of value to all sports. Jogging on the spot (running without lifting the knees too high or moving forward) is very much favoured by Americans and can easily be included in the daily routine. Skipping with a rope can also be done in a limited space.

Weight lifting or training produces good conditioning of the body and increases the working efficiency of the muscles. Basic weight-resisting exercises are nowadays considered an important part of modern training – not in order to become a weight lifter but to increase muscle power, stamina and cardio-vascular fitness. Athletes who move quickly – such as short-distance runners, footballers and tennis players – should confine their amount of weight lifting to about 20 lb. Discus throwers and shot putters should gradually work up to as much as 80 lb.

Both the Swedes and the Germans developed *interval running* just before the Second World War. The Swedish idea was the more aesthetic. They believed that by training in picturesque settings with varying terrains they could combine fast bursts of speed with relaxing slow periods to suit the contours of the land. The German method was more precise: short bursts of running at speed with recovery periods.

Circuit training is a form of interval training nowadays popular in the United States, although it has been used with success in England for years. It consists of a series of exercises done at various stages. There are about ten different routines (a rope climb or ladder walking, for instance) according to the equipment available. The circuit is performed as fast as possible doing each routine a given number of times before passing on to the next. When the athlete has mastered one circuit, the number of circuits is increased and all rounds are against time. As he improves, his time is reduced until he reaches a maximum speed at which point the degree of fitness possible for him is said to have been achieved.

These methods have been standardised and included in most plans of general training so that there are specific lengths of time for speed and recovery. Most sports require the athlete to be able to run effectively. If, however, a miler is being trained, he will run a quarter of a mile at speed, a slow quarter, a fast quarter and a slow, gradually increasing the fast quarters until he is approximating four minutes for his mile.

Alford, the athletic trainer who was the famous pre-war miler, has said that present-day athletes train at least five times harder than their counterparts before the war. For top athletes there is no such thing as a complete season of rest; they train almost all the year round even during the off season. This concentrated training is probably the reason for the breaking of records each year.

Mental Preparation

Mental and psychological fitness are necessary to reach the pinnacle of any sport. When an athlete, capable of reaching the heights, has an off day he will usually excuse it by saying, 'I was simply not able to concentrate.' This may be due to some personal worry or to the fact that his morale had somehow been lowered; sometimes it is caused by a belief that he will fail, or by a boredom caused by over-training, sometimes even by economic worries. On the other hand, concentration comes from many sources and some professional sportsmen are said to be able to concentrate more effort into winning when the prize is bigger. Dedication to the sport, the will to win and even fear of losing can all play their part.

When a player is able to cast all his worries on to his coach he is then able to apply himself totally to the event.

Preparation for Special Events

By the end of the sixth week of training the athlete has already taken part actively in his sport but he probably has some special future event in mind. He may be close to one-hundred-per-cent fitness but still needs just that extra impetus. He should try to keep himself at the level he has reached until the time comes to raise himself to the very summit of training.

Obviously, with every sport, the final toughening up period will be different. Each athlete and his trainer will know best how to reach maximum fitness without going over the top into over-training and staleness.

However, while at one time it was considered that the only way to overcome staleness was to rest, it is now believed to be better to work through the barren period and get over it, and that there is no such thing as over-training.

Preparation for Specific Skills

Towards the end of the second week those who are training for special sports – golf, tennis, boxing, sculling, show jumping, swimming, athletics, football, cricket and a great many others – start doing specific activities connected with their sport. By this time any early stiffness should have worn off. Hot baths and rubbing with a coarse towel should ease any pain but in the case of excessive stiffness the level of exercise should not be increased until the stiffness has worn off.

Training Exercises

Bertie Mee, who guided Arsenal to many triumphs, devised a set of exercises for his players which would be good preparation for any sport though 'Soccer is the most popular game in the world', he declares firmly. 'Soccer never stands still.' He also has certain tests for fitness.

> Soccer is a game which takes a heavy toll of weak muscles [he says]. If you think of a muscle as a piece of elastic . . . stretch it out to full length and let it snap together and it will return to its original length. If you stretch it to its full length many times, each time releasing it gradually, it will eventually lengthen. That is what we try to do with our stretch exercises. In the beginning these exercises were devised for rehabilitation. Sometimes a player, eager to return to the game, would claim full recovery, but when we tested him we found that he still favoured the injured side. We then put him on a full course of exercises which would build up the injured muscle. Then it seemed possible that if these muscles were stretched and strengthened before play the injuries might not occur and this has proved to be the case. We reduced the injuries on the field by fifty per cent. These injuries were mostly soft tissue injuries to hamstrings, calves, quadriceps and adductors. You must have full extensibility before soft tissue injuries can be considered recovered or they will break down again.

In testing the hip, if the injured hip is not one-hundred-per-cent fit the weight is not fully taken on the injured foot, the hip coming up slightly. Again, when sitting on the heels and leaning back on the hands, if the hip is not completely fit the exercise will not be done equally on both sides and the trunk will tend to lean towards the good side.

When testing hamstrings in a forward bend with stiff knees, the player is apt to touch the toe only on the uninjured side, favouring the injured hamstrings.

Here are the fitness exercises:

Exercises for the rectus femorus (the middle of the thigh in front), which is the kicking muscle. Feet wide apart, make a slight lunge, bending the knee outward. Then lunge on the opposite side.

Exercise for the groin. Put one foot on a chair with the leg at right angles to the body. Bend towards the chair feeling the stretch on the inside of the thighs from groin to knee. Change legs and repeat.

Exercise for the calf. Without shoes, heels flat, knees straight, stand about a foot from a wall, hands supporting the body at shoulder height, then lean forward, feeling the stretch of the muscles all up the back of the calf and thigh. Push upright again and repeat. Knees must be straight.

2

Injuries Common to Most Sports and their First-Aid

Many injuries in sport vary in their original cause and severity but have similar symptoms and require comparable treatment.

First-Aid: Objectives and Essentials

1. Protection and support of the injured part so that the condition is not allowed to be aggravated.

2. Removal of all tight articles of clothing which could interfere with breathing or heart action.

3. Control of swelling caused by injury with firm bandaging. Application of ice packs and elevation of the injured part if possible.

4. The treatment of general conditions such as shock and unconsciousness.

5. In compound wounds the arrest of haemorrhage by finger pressure, firm bandaging, ice packs if available – a cold sponge if not – and the use of a tourniquet only if absolutely necessary to stop excessive blood flow. The application of a sterile dressing should be used to prevent further contamination. If firmly applied it will also stop bleeding.

6. Urgent and quick transport to medical care and treatment.

7. In the case of sun or heatstroke the person should be protected from the heat as much as possible and cold compresses with ice applied to the head and any constrictive clothing loosened.

8. If an epileptic fit is suspected, a firm object, such as a spoon, pen or wooden stick should be placed between the teeth to prevent biting of the tongue, and dentures removed.

Unconsciousness

In active sports loss of consciousness is most likely to be caused by concussion as the result of a head injury. A fracture of the skull may also produce unconsciousness as can happen in motor-car or motor-cycle races, falls or kicks from a horse, hitting solid objects while skiing, by being kicked by a boot in rugby football or hit on the face or head by a fast bowler at cricket.

If the surface of the skull is pushed into the brain substance it is called a depressed fracture. If it occurs in the motor area (the cerebral cortex) Jacksonian fits may result – that is, biting the tongue, contracting muscles and passing urine and faeces.

In boxing, unconsciousness may occur about three times in a hundred bouts, caused by one or many blows to the head, or by the head striking the floor of the ring. If the boxer is hit on the jaw with sufficient force, this force is transferred to the base of the brain from the point of the jaw, causing minute haemorrhages in the brain substance and unconsciousness. This could also happen in other sports.

If the cause of the unconsciousness is not immediately obvious, preliminary diagnosis should be attempted. Slow pulse, laboured respiration and vomiting indicate cranial pressure. Bleeding from the nose or mouth or ears could denote fracture at the base of the skull. The lids should be lifted and the eyes examined. Constricted pupils may imply drug addiction or disease affecting the central nervous system. Dilated pupils, which often occur in the unconscious state, may also appear after a heart attack (cardiac arrest). Unequal pupils – one dilated, one constricted – may indicate unequal pressure in the skull on the two sides following a head injury or a stroke.

Other causes of unconsciousness are sunstroke, when the pulse will be strong and rapid, the temperature high, face red, pupils dilated and breathing laboured; and heat exhaustion, when the face is pale, skin cold and perspiring, temperature low and breathing shallow.

Less likely in sports but still possible are diabetic comas, heart attacks, epileptic fits and, on rare occasions, death.

Since 1931 fewer than thirty soccer players have died from head injuries, a small proportion of the many who play football. Some deaths were attributed to heading the ball, others to a possible collision with a boot after a fall.

In boxing, death has occurred very rarely despite the possibility of severe head injury. Dr Adrian Whiteside, Medical Officer of the British Boxing Board of Control, has said:'Because of the less stringent medical controls there is more risk of head injury in football than in boxing. If a boxer is knocked unconscious he is stopped from competing, kept under observation and prevented from sparring for at least twenty-one days. If a footballer is concussed, out come the smelling-salts, wet sponge and on he goes.' Certainly even momentary loss of consciousness is an indication that the player must come off the field.

Soft Tissue Injuries

The soft tissues of the body consist of the following from the surface inwards: (i) the skin; (ii) fibrous tissues and fat called the subcutaneous tissue; (iii) the muscle layers; (iv) arteries, veins, nerves with lymph channels and lymph glands. These are distinct from the hard bony structures which go to make up the skeleton.

Initially almost all athletic injuries affect the soft tissue whatever other structures are involved. Bruising of the soft tissues, a pulled or torn muscle, strains, sprains of joint structures account for about two thirds of the total. These, however trivial they may appear, should be taken seriously and correctly treated if undesirable after-effects are to be prevented. The aim of treatment is to restore the sportsman to the same condition of good health, both structurally and functionally, he was in before the accident.

A direct blow causes bruising of the soft tissues (a contusion). This may result in damage to the surface of the skin, crushing of the blood vessels, nerves, and even death of some tissue cells, and, if severe enough, may also result in injury to the bony structures such as fractures.

An *indirect* injury can cause tearing of the tissues on one side of the limb such as a strained or torn ligament, a pulled muscle or strain, whereas those of the opposite side suffer *direct* trauma by the bony structures being forced on to soft tissue structures causing compression and contusion (bruising).

When the skin is unbroken, it is considered a closed or simple wound; when the skin is broken, it should be treated as an open or compound wound.

SOFT TISSUE INJURIES: CLOSED OR SIMPLE
With a heavy blow, considerable tissue destruction may take place. The

36

damage is below the skin surface and swelling and pain will result. Its severity will depend on how deep the damage has gone. If small blood vessels are broken there will be discoloration of the skin – bruising (contusion). If the larger blood vessels are involved, blood may collect and form a collection of blood in the soft tissue (a haematoma). This is the result of the escape of blood from torn or crushed blood vessels in the soft tissue.

The injury may occur to a joint. A joint consists of a capsule which is divided into two parts: the fibrous capsule and the synovial membrane. The fibrous capsule holds the bones together while the synovial membrane secretes fluid to oil the joint. When the joint is damaged the synovial membrane is stimulated, the joint swells and the structures are tender and painful on movement. If the swelling of the joint takes place immediately after the accident a blood vessel may have been torn in the joint itself and bleeding into the joint has occurred causing a haemarthrosis.

First-Aid. Cold compresses or an ice pack will help reduce the swelling. Firm support by a pad of lint with layers of wool over it, held by a firm compression bandage, with elevation of the limb, is advisable. If the damage is not deep and the player can return to his sport, the area should be supported by a firm bandage or strapping, if possible over stockinet.

OPEN SOFT TISSUE WOUNDS

In these the skin is broken or abrased, either by rubbing or scraping, by a direct cut or a blow, say, from a boot or a contact blow. The main thing is to prevent infection.

First-Aid. Bleeding must be controlled, then a disinfectant applied if available and the wound covered with a bandage or Band-aid. Nothing embedded in the wound, not even dirt, should be removed at this stage as haemorrhage might result.

If the wound in the skin is insignificant, no treatment for a clean cut may be necessary beyond changing the bandage and applying fresh disinfectant. However, there may also be underlying damage which should be treated, as in closed soft tissue injuries. If dirt or other substances are in the wound, treatment must be carried out by a doctor, preferably in the emergency department of a hospital. He may have to give an antibiotic and possibly anti-tetanus serum or toxoid.

Strains

A strain is an injury to a muscle, tendon or ligament resulting from overuse or misuse which causes excessive stretching and can be *mild*, *moderate* or *severe*. For example, strains can be caused by lifting heavy objects or weights while in an unbalanced position. Strains of the forearm muscles and tendons may be caused by a repetitive movement performed incorrectly. These may start by being mild. For instance, at tennis or golf the player may gradually develop a strained elbow. In football an acute strain or even the rupture of a muscle with swelling and haematoma formation may occur if the player tries to kick a ball which is blocked. This throws unexpected strain on one of the quadriceps muscles in front of the thigh with resulting injury. Inflammation of the muscle on the back of the upper arm (triceps) can occur in a pitcher in baseball if he is over-ambitious or under-trained, possibly eventually resulting in a complete rupture.

First-Aid
Mild Strain. Support with bandage or strapping. The player can probably continue his sport (see pp. 46–7).

Moderate Strain. The player will have swelling and pain when carrying out movements. He may have to come off the field if he cannot function normally without pain. At first, support with a removable bandage over wool is advocated. Do not strap unless he is able to go back into play.

Severe Strain. If the player cannot take weight on his lower limbs, or hold a bat, racket, ball or whatever, or if the damage is in the upper extremities, he must come off the field and the limb must be supported and the weight taken off if in a lower extremity.

Secondary Treatment. For mild or moderate strains, contrast baths or ice packs can be given. This consists of bathing the injured part alternatively with hot and cold water for about ten to fifteen minutes. In cases of severe strain it must be ascertained if a fracture or a dislocation has taken place, in which case the player must go to hospital. The damaged limb must be supported by whatever type of splint is available. In the case of a lower-limb injury, sticks or crutches should be used; for an upper arm, a sling.

Sprains

These occur through sudden violent wrenching or twisting of a joint, causing tendons and ligaments to stretch and even rupture, such as could occur in skiing or football.

There is usually a rapid swelling of the joint structures and the injured part cannot be moved without pain; there will be evidence of contusion and bruising of the tissues almost immediately.

First-Aid. The injured part should be protected and supported so that the condition is not allowed to be aggravated. Control of traumatic effusion should be ensured by firm bandaging and the positioning of the injured part in elevation if possible. At this stage immobilisation should be as complete as possible.

Secondary Treatment. The player should be given quick transport to medical care and treatment, preferably in the emergency department of a hospital.

Subluxation

A subluxation is a partial dislocation of the bony structures of a joint, usually within range of normal movement. The subluxation may be momentary, with the opposing joint surface held by the capsule or by muscle spasm in a slightly abnormal position, the joint springing back into position of its own accord. If this occurs, first-aid should be the same as in the case of a sprained joint, with protection and support, though there may be some soreness or stiffness with home treatment later.

Dislocation

A dislocation is total displacement of the bones composing a joint outside its normal range of movement and position in the joint as, for example, when the shoulder 'comes out of joint' due either to direct or indirect violence. A direct injury, such as a blow on the shoulder, may cause the head of the bone of the upper arms to be thrust downwards against the joint capsule, pushing it out of place.

Dislocation of the shoulder due to indirect injury may occur when the player falls but tries to stem the fall with his hand or elbow.

Other vulnerable joints are those of the outer end of the collar bone, the elbow, ankle, fingers and, occasionally, the hip and knee.

A complete dislocation may cause tearing of the ligaments and make the joint unstable. Once this has happened there is a danger of recurrence.

There may be deformity of the joint before reduction with symptoms similar to a severe sprain: swelling and pain and limitation of movement. A dislocated bone may cause pressure on nerves and paralysis of the surrounding muscles or even pressure on blood vessels. Dislocation of a spinal vertebra may compress the spinal cord. Dislocation of the elbow joint may press on blood vessels with a resulting blueness and coldness of the hand.

Where a recurrent dislocation takes place it is likely to be due to improper healing of the previously torn capsule and ligaments with stretching, weakness and wasting of the corresponding muscles.

First-Aid. Dislocations must be reduced – put back in the socket – with great care. This may be accomplished immediately they happen and in any sport where they are likely to occur it is as well for the person in charge to know how it should be done. The bones must be pulled completely apart so as to stretch the joint capsule. Then, with the bony ends in alignment, twist or pressure on the displaced end of the distal bone will cause it to fall into place. Reduction of the joints of the fingers may be accomplished by the player himself or the referee or coach, but dislocations of major joints are better left to the medical practitioner as they may be complicated by a fracture, injury to ligaments, nerves and blood vessels. Speedy removal to surgical care is essential as reduction by a surgeon under full general anaesthesia may be necessary.

Fractures: Simple

This is a fracture of a bone where the skin is not broken. There is no wound and it can sometimes be mistaken for a sprain or strain unless there is obvious deformity. The force can be direct – where the blow falls at the point of breakage – or indirect where the injury is received at some distance from the break. This may happen, for example, where a twisting movement of the ankle in snow skiing goes beyond a sprain and results in a broken bone or bones of the ankle. A fall on the hand, apart from causing fractures at the wrist (radius and ulna) through direct injury, can also produce a fracture of bones higher up (radius and humerus) through indirect injury with possible dislocation of the elbow and shoulder.

First-Aid. Protection and support of the injured part so that the condition is not allowed to be aggravated. If there is no displacement of bones, simple bandaging may be all that is necessary. However, the support of the injured part may need more than bandaging, especially where there is obvious deformity and the fractured ends seem to move about. In these cases splints may have to be applied before the part is moved and urgent removal to hospital is advisable because of the danger of complications to blood vessels and nerves.

Fractures: Compound

In a compound or open fracture the bone may be sticking through the skin, making an open wound which may be oozing blood. To be called a compound fracture, the break in the skin must lead down to the fractured bones.

First-Aid. Cut or tear clothing away from the wound. Treat bleeding and prevent contamination by lightly placing a sterile dressing over the area. Splint before moving, even if only in the most primitive manner.

Fractures: Skull

The skull may be broken or cracked or there may be a depressed fracture in which the skull is broken and the fragments of bone are embedded in the brain.

First-Aid. The person in charge need not try to distinguish between fractures and concussion since the first-aid treatment is the same for both injuries. If the face is normal or red, the head should be slightly raised. If the face is pale, the head should be kept level. Avoid unnecessary handling and keep the patient warm. Control external bleeding with a sterile pad but do not use antiseptics or remove anything from the wound. Turn the head slightly to one side if blood or mucus collects in the throat or mouth. If breathing stops, institute artificial respiration immediately.

Fractures: Neck or Spine

Remember there are three parts of the mobile spine: (i) Upper (cervical); (ii) Middle (dorsal or thoracic); (iii) Lower (lumbar). A fracture in any part of the back is serious, though fortunately rare in most sports. It can, however, occur in such sports as motor racing, motor cycling, National Hunt racing, fox hunting, diving and sometimes in winter sports. If the spinal cord suffers damage, death may occur. If the upper cervical spine is involved, total paralysis is probable if the sportsman survives. If in the lower cervical spine, paralysis of the upper extremity can happen; or if in the dorsal and lumbar spine it may be the trunk and lower extremities which are affected.

First-Aid can cause more harm than the original damage if great care is not taken. The person suspected of a fractured spine should not be moved even to change the head to a more comfortable position. Apart from paralysis, there may be loss of sensation in the area affected by that part of the spinal cord involved and pain at the site of fracture may be severe, particularly on even the slightest movement.

If it is absolutely necessary that the patient be moved before the arrival of the physician, at least four strong men should help in the transfer. One of them should hold the head steady on a line with the spine and not allow it to rotate or bend sideways. Two others may then lift the body and the fourth steady the legs. He must be placed on a flat surface, such as a door. His arms should be placed at his sides and his head and arms immobilised by the use of hard pillows or sandbags. The injured person's head must not be lifted.

A new type of stretcher has been devised in Australia which is made to fit and support the injured person when he is lying on the ground. The framework of the stretcher is placed around the patient and the adjustable plastic straps are fitted under him and held attached to the framework of the stretcher on two corresponding sides. The patient can be transported prone or supine.

Fractures: Stress or Fatigue

These are caused by a constant strain on bones at a point where maximum stress occurs. In walking events the bones of the foot may fracture. A whipping force is applied to the bone resulting in the stress fracture –

sometimes called a 'fatigue fracture'. These have been reported in athletes of different types such as skaters, long-distance walkers and cricketers. The bones at the base of the toes (metatarsal) and those of the lower leg (tibia and fibula) are the most common sites.

First-Aid. This is similar to the treatment of simple fractures once diagnosed, but they may be mistaken, on the field, for a sprain and an X-ray may be needed to prove the break. Protection and support of the injured part by suitable bandaging and strapping is the most effective treatment and, of course, rest.

Fractures: the Use of Splints

Before applying splints, ascertain whether nerve function and the blood supply appear to be involved – as shown by paralysis of the muscles or severe alteration of the colour of the limb below the fracture. If there is also gross displacement, straighten the distal part of the limb with traction. This may produce reduction with immediate release of pressure on the nerves and blood vessels.

Traction, in a severely angulated fracture, may be carried out by gently but firmly holding the limb furthest from the fracture, that is, the hand or foot, and straightening the bent arm or leg. This procedure may give momentary pain but afterwards gives considerable relief.

IMPROVISED SPLINTS
In an emergency the crudest of improvised splints can be made from bits of wood, metal, cardboard or newspaper fastened on with bandages or straps. Pillows can be excellent for immobilising the ankle and foot and can be fastened around with safety pins. The splint should, if possible, be long enough to extend over the joints above and below the fracture. Preferably, commercially-made splints should be kept on hand by those in charge of sports where fractures are possible or likely as these are designed for specific injuries and are more effective than the improvised affairs.

They include padded boards, air splints, wire ladder splints, foam rubber splints, arthropads, plastic or foam rubber collars, backboards and others. The aim in every case is to immobilise the joints above and below as well. In first-aid for broken leg or ankle bones, the splints can be placed over clothing and without even removing shoes, provided the skin is not broken.

Air Splints. These are among the most useful to keep on hand as they are easy to store. They come in several sizes and it is as well to study the instructions which come with them before the need for using them arises. They consist of a double-walled plastic tube and some of them have zippers. They are inflated by mouth and the only danger is that they will be blown up too hard. It should be possible to indent the 'balloon' with the thumb after it is inflated. They give a good uniform pressure.

For use with a broken bone in the arm or leg the person doing the first-aid should put the deflated splint on his own arm and gently draw the hand or foot into the bag while supporting the break with the other hand. Then inflate.

Small air splints are useful for damaged hands with broken bones and soft tissue injury. The fingers should be slightly curved and kept that way by means of a roll of gauze placed in the palm. The air splint will immobilise the hand yet give gentle compression only to the injured tissue.

Wire Ladder Splints padded with gamgee. These are particularly good for use with a fracture of the forearm as they can be bent at the elbow. The hand rests on one end, the other supporting the upper arm – the joint above and below the fracture. The whole is then supported by a sling.

Hexcelite Splints. These are made from a plastic material which, when heated either in an oven or in hot water, can be moulded and cut to shape on the patient. They are self-adhesive when warm, set within ten minutes and are light and comfortable to wear.

Slings

The usual way to wear a sling is to suspend it round the neck. Universal slings, which should be part of any first-aid kit for sportsmen, should never be hung round the neck as this exerts undue pressure on the neck muscles. The sling should permit the weight of the injured arm to be carried by the opposite shoulder. The Bourbon sling and the Cradle arm sling are others which follow this principle. Occasionally a collar-and-cuff sling is allowed in children.

Application of a Tourniquet

If possible, use of a tourniquet should be avoided as firm pressure from a pad of wool and firm bandage will in many cases be sufficient to control bleeding. Soft, flat material at least three or four inches wide should be used if it is absolutely essential, and this can be made out of a triangular bandage folded into six or eight layers three or four inches wide. A rubber tube, a blood-pressure cuff or a long handkerchief can be used. The material should be wrapped twice around the extremity and half-knotted at a level proximal to the point of bleeding. A stick or similar object placed on top of the flat knot should be secured by tying the end of the bandage in a square (reef) knot. Twist the stick to tighten the tourniquet until the bleeding stops – no more. Loosen the tourniquet gently at ten-minute intervals.

Tourniquets have been known to cause damage to nerves and blood vessels and, if left on for too long, they may result in loss of an arm or leg. Therefore, when the patient is taken away for medical attention, the tourniquet should be in plain sight and as an additional precaution 'TK' should be written on his forehead. It should also be pointed out to the ambulance attendent or medical staff that a tourniquet has been applied.

When a Player Must Leave the Field

One of the most responsible and hardest decisions for the coach, referee or umpire to make is when it would be safe for the injured sportsman to return to his sport after treatment. In some cases – where he has been unconscious or suffered broken limbs – the answer is obvious. In other cases there may be doubtful factors, not the least of which may be the player's own feelings in the matter which may have to be overridden. The man in charge will have to know his athletes and their characters. Some may be too brave and insist on carrying on even when this is inadvisable. Others may be just the reverse – afraid to retire in case they are thought to be cowards. Others may be so careful of themselves that they may wish to come off when in fact no harm would come to them if they had stayed on.

If it is a team game there are also the other players to be considered and certain questions must be asked. Are reserves allowed? If not, is the game so important to the team that the safety of one player must be risked? Is there a future event for which the injured player must be at his best?

This last question also applies to sports where the player is on his own: athletics, swimming, tennis and golf, among others. Even here there might be a situation in, say, the Olympic Games, where if one retires the others forfeit the medal or the chance of a medal. This has happened in show jumping and eventing.

The following chart may help with difficult decisions.

To Show When a Player Should Leave the Field or Could Remai

Condition	State or Symptoms	Must Leave/May Remain		First-Aid
Loss of consciousness	Heart attack. Possible concussion. Diabetic coma	Always	Never	Make sure air passage free. Send for ambulanc
Concussion	Fast pulse, unequal pupils, unconsciousness, stertorous breathing, irregular pulse, urinating or defaecating	Always	Never	As above. See he does n swallow tongue
Winded	Gasping for breath, clutching stomach. Possible whiplash		Yes, if no other injury	Sponge with cold water
Broken bones simple: closed, no wound	Undue mobility of the bones with deformity and loss of function	Always	Never	Immobilise limb, straighten and use temporary splint. No stimulants. Send for ambulance
Broken bones: compound	As above with open wound to site of fracture or ends protruding through open wound	Always	Never	As above with sterile pad of gauze on wound

46

Broken bones: neck or spine	Possible paralysis	Always	Never	If necessary to move off field five people needed. Use door as stretcher, sandbags to steady head. Send for ambulance
Subluxations	Joint slightly out of socket, some pain	Possibly	Yes, if joint snaps back and is not too painful	If finger, player can help himself. Shoulder or hip: pull hand or foot until slight click
Dislocations	Obvious symptoms shoulder, hip or knee. Unless simple positioning reduces, finger dislocations may be reduced by player or coach	Always	Never	Joint should be protected by strapping or splintage. Refer to hospital. Bind with Scotch tape or Prestotape. Refer to hospital
Sprains: severe	Severe swelling with great pain or joint instability. Inability to take weight on lower extremities or grasp with fingers	Always	Never	Cold compresses, ice packs or sprays. Refer to hospital for X-ray
Sprains: mild	Little pain or joint instability, no effusion	If game important, can return to play		Support with strapping or bandaging
Open wounds without fracture		Depends on severity. *No* if dirty; *yes* if slight after first-aid		Arrest bleeding, protect and support. Disinfect wound. If no previous anti-tetanus injection refer to hospital, if wound is dirty
Closed contusions with bruising	If deep in a muscle with pain on movement	Always	Never	Ice packs, firm support and refer to hospital
Minor	Surface bruise without abrasion		Can return to play after first-aid	Attention on field with sponge or sprey and suitable support

47

First-Aid Kit

Adhesive tape, several widths
Rolls of Elastoplast bandages
Sterile pads in sterile containers
4 × 4 gauge roller bandages
Ammonia in capsules or smelling salts for restoring consciousness
Liquid ammonia for stings or bites where likely to happen
Burn ointment where likely to happen
Tube analgesic cream or balm; can also be used for sunburn
Vaseline
Material for tourniquets
Scissors
Thermometer
Eye cup and wash
Universal slings
Safety pins
Splinter forceps
70 per cent alcohol as antiseptic or iodine
Aspirin
Salt tablets for cramp caused by dehydration if likely
Ice bag if ice available
Roll of cottonwool
Talcum powder for feet or massage
Surgical soap for cleaning wounds when advisable
Sponge and bucket for field work if any
Oil of cloves for toothache
Tube or bottle of adhesive tape remover
Telephone number of doctor, ambulance and/or hospital

Comparative Injuries in Various Sports

In a series of 6,057 consecutive sports injuries compiled by Dr Otto Johanson

Skiing	1,784	Wrestling	116
Football	1,320	Boxing	100
Gymnastics	622	Athletics	90
Swimming and Diving	523	Cross-country running	57
Handball	393	Tennis	30
Skating	363	Other Sports	245
Tobogganing	279		6,057
Hockey, field and ice	135		

Tips from the American Academy of Orthopaedic Surgeons

Certain memory joggers devised by this group of doctors are useful for the referee, touch judge, umpire, spectator or player who, with little knowledge or training in first-aid, is called upon in an emergency to render treatment.

UNCONSCIOUSNESS

To remember the causes, use the five vowels: A – Apoplexy (stroke); E – Epilepsy; I – Injury; O – Opium or other drugs; U – Uremia (toxicity because of kidney failure or other disturbed metabolic states such as diabetes mellitis).

In considering an athlete on the field of play, A (stroke) may be caused by heat. Injury, of course, is the most likely cause of unconsciousness.

Another simple diagnostic test is whether the skin is red, white or blue. In sunstroke or diabetic coma the face is always red. In any type of shock, heat exhaustion, freezing or bleeding the face is white. With suffocation or electric shock the fingertips are blue.

For cardio-pulmonary resuscitation the letters A, B and C are to be remembered: Airway, Breathing and Circulation. The *Airway* must be opened and any obstruction removed; the *Breathing* must be restored by artificial ventilation; the *Circulation* must be restored by external cardiac compression.

The American Academy recommends the following points for action on the scene of serious injuries:

1. Remove patient to situation of safety.
2. Restrain other players or bystanders from crowding.
3. Obtain assistance from qualified volunteers only.
4. Avoid assuming duties of the police if these are present.

Red, White and Blue Signs of Unconsciousness*

CONDITION	USUAL SIGNS						OTHER SIGNS	MANAGEMENT	
	Unconscious?	Face	Skin	Pulse	Breathing	Eyes		Special	General

Red Unconsciousness

CONDITION	Unconscious?	Face	Skin	Pulse	Breathing	Eyes	OTHER SIGNS	Special	General
SUNSTROKE (HEAT STROKE)	If severe	Red	Dry and very hot	Strong and rapid	Laboured	Pupils dilated	Headache, high temperature, sweating ceases	Apply cold applications to head. Cool body. Keep in shade	In every case of red unconsciousness: 1. Watch breathing carefully. Artificial ventilation may be necessary 2. Keep patient lying down 3. Apply cold application to head 4. Give nothing by mouth while unconscious 5. Get ready to transport
STROKE	Usually	Red, pale, or normal	Normal; later may be cool and moist	Strong and slow	Snoring	Pupils sometimes unequal	Paralysis, twitching, or convulsions		
DRUNKENNESS	Sometimes	Red, pale, or normal	Normal; later may be cool and moist	Strong; later weak	Deep or shallow	Pupils normal or dilated; eyeballs red	No paralysis		
SKULL FRACTURE AND CONCUSSION	Sometimes	Red, pale, or normal	Normal; later may be cool and moist	Strong and slow; or rapid and weak	Deep or shallow	Pupils may be unequal	Evidence of blow; bleeding at nose, ear, or mouth	Cover wound with sterile dressing. Apply no antiseptics to wound	
EPILEPSY	Yes; later consciousness or deep sleep	Pale; later bluish-red; then normal				Eyes rolled upwards	Hoarse cry; bites tongue; makes convulsive muscular movements; falls down	Prevent patient from injuring himself. No restraint of convulsive muscular movements. Rest after convulsions	
DIABETIC COMA	Always	Red	Dry	Weak, rapid	Air hunger	Eyeballs soft	Acetone odor		

White Unconsciousness

CONDITION	Unconscious?	Face	Skin	Pulse	Breathing	Eyes	OTHER SIGNS	Special	General
BLEEDING	Sometimes	Pale	Cold and perspiring	Rapid and weak	Shallow	Pupils normal or dilated	Blood usually obvious; may cough or spit up blood	Stop bleeding; if bleeding internally give no stimulant dress wound	In every case of white unconsciousness: 1. Watch breathing carefully. Artificial ventilation may be necessary 2. Keep patient's head down 3. Loosen clothing 4. Give nothing by mouth while unconscious 5. Get ready to transport
SHOCK	Sometimes	Pale	Cold and perspiring	Rapid and weak	Shallow	Pupils normal or dilated	Restless	Keep warm (avoid chilling) and keeping down with feet slightly elevated	
HEAT EXHAUSTION	Sometimes	Pale	Cold and perspiring	Rapid and weak	Shallow	Pupils normal or dilated	Nausea, vomiting, low temperature, cramps	Remove to shade or cool place. Give salt solution when patient can drink	
FAINTING	Briefly	Pale	Cold and	Rapid	Shallow	Pupils	Physical weakness	Give fresh air. Keep head	

	Unconscious?	Face	Skin	Pulse	Breathing	Eyes	Special	General
POISONS	Sometimes	Tongue, lips, or mouth may be burned or stained					Pain in stomach, nausea, vomiting, cramps; evidence of poison container	Give artificial ventilation if breathing stops
INSULIN SHOCK	Sometimes	Pale	Moist	Normal	Shallow	Pupils normal or dilated		Administer sweets
FREEZING	Sometimes	White or greyish white	Cold				Depression	Remove from surroundings and place in warm room. Artificial ventilation if breathing has stopped
CONVULSIONS	Yes; later falls asleep	Pale; later blue					Extreme restlessness; convulsive muscular movements; body may become stiff or bend backward	**Don't try to stop convulsions.** Keep harmful objects out of the way. Try to prevent from biting tongue by placing pad between teeth

Blue Unconsciousness

	Unconscious?	Face	Skin	Pulse	Breathing	Eyes	Special	General
SUFFOCATION	Yes	Pale lips; fingertips blue	Cold and perspiring	Rapid and weak; sometimes absent	Stopped	Pupils normal or dilated	Insure airway. Start artificial ventilation immediately	**In every case of blue unconsciousness:** 1. Watch breathing carefully. Artificial ventilation may be necessary 2. Keep patient lying down 3. Give nothing by mouth while unconscious 4. Get ready to transport
ELECTRIC SHOCK	Sometimes	Lips pale; fingertips blue	Cold and perspiring	May be absent	Stopped	Pupils large	Mechanism of injury seen	Remove from source. Give cardiopulmonary resuscitation at once if in cardiac arrest

*Reprinted with the kind permission of the American Academy of Orthopaedic Surgeons.

51

3
First-Aid in Specific Sports

Athletics: Running, High Jump, Long Jump, Cross-Country Running, Discus Throwing, Javelin Throwing, Shot-Putting

STRAINS, PULLS AND TEARS

All runners can get strains of calf muscles or hamstrings which produce muscle spasms that may, in turn, lead to severe tears. These can make the runner go down as if shot in the leg. An ankle strain can also be caused by the athlete running flat-footed, the stress being thrown on one of the lower leg bones (fibula) about six inches from the lower end.

Pulled muscles are the most common form of injury for sprinters, especially rupture of muscle fibres in the thigh, hamstrings and calf muscles.

First-Aid for strains, pulls or tears consists of removing the athlete from the track immediately, applying ice packs and giving him support for the injured joint or muscle. Recurrence is probable unless complete healing takes place with return of full muscle power.

Similar treatment should be given to stress fracture of the bones at the base of the toes (metatarsal) or in the lower leg (fibula)

CUTS AND BRUISES

In modern competitive running, jostling is so common that a runner may fall. Contusions, bruises, abrasions may result on any part of his body or

52

he may suffer from cuts from the spikes in other competitors' shoes.

First-Aid. As well as normal precautions against infection – bathing with mild antiseptic and bandaging with sterile gauze – it may be necessary for an athlete to have anti-tetanus or toxoid injections if he has not already had them.

SORENESS OF THE FEET AND SHINS
In long-distance or cross-country running a foot may strike the ground five thousand times in an hour. Sorbo soles inside the shoes, which should be half a size larger than usual, often prevent any soreness on the under-side of the foot.

With long-distance running over hard roads or surfaces or, in orienteering, over rough territory which may include ditches to be jumped, hills to be climbed, gates to be surmounted, shin soreness is a real problem, though it may not make itself felt until the next day when every muscle feels like brittle cardboard.

First-Aid. The soreness can be relieved, along with stiffness, by taking a long hot bath alternated with ice-cold sponging while still in the bath. Additions to the bath of sea salt, seaweed preparations or Radox or Fynnon Spa salts are of some help.

BRUISED HEEL
An injury specific to long jumpers is a bruised heel as they often come down hard on the take-off board.

First-Aid. There is no specific first-aid for this condition except to stop jumping until the condition recovers through time, physiotherapy and other medical treatment. Cushioning the heel with Sorbo rubber is often advised to aid recovery and ensure against repetition.

PULLED TENDO-ACHILLES
A long jumper can suffer pain from a pulled tendo-achilles greater than the injury would seem to warrant. The pain is usually deep in the tendon and there is a small thickening or lump two inches above the insertion of the heel bone.

First-Aid. Considerable relief is gained from Elastoplast wound round the ankle and lower leg at the site of the injury.

PAIN IN THE TOES

High jumpers may get a radiating pain in the second, third and fourth toes, due to landing badly, caused by a thickening (false neuroma) on the digital nerves.

First-Aid. A Sorbo rubber metatarsal pad can reduce pain but, if the relief is not adequate, minor surgery to remove the thickened segment of the nerve may be recommended.

SPRAINED ANKLE OR SHOULDER

A high jumper may also get a foot in the wrong position for landing and rick his ankle, causing muscles to be strained, sprained or torn. If he lands on his shoulder he may bruise and contuse the shoulder or sprain the joints.

First-Aid. Rest and elevation for the ankle, a universal or improvised sling for the arm until medical attention and physiotherapy can be given.

'THROWER'S SHOULDER'

Discus throwers, javelin throwers and shot-putters may get a so-called 'thrower's shoulder' or rotation strains of the back.

First-Aid. No first-aid can help, but the athlete *must* stop throwing. A doctor may decide to give injections of a local anaesthetic and hydro-cortisone as this often brings relief of pain.

STRAINED ELBOW

The inside of the elbow (medial collateral ligament) can be strained and the tip of the bone of the elbow (olecranon) can be strained by throwing round-arm.

First-Aid. Rest is the best treatment for elbow injuries though even after they have become symptom-free the injury tends to recur with the return to throwing.

DISABILITIES CAUSED TO ATHLETES BY EXCESSES OF CLIMATE

Heat cramps, heat exhaustion and heat stroke can affect athletes in very hot weather.

Heat Cramps

Painful spasms of muscles in the legs and sometimes the arms are usually due to lack of salt which has been excreted by sweating.

First-Aid. Cramps are usually relieved quite quickly if a solution of salt is drunk – a level teaspoon to a quart of water. Salt tablets are also effective and competitive athletes are allowed to carry them on long-distance runs.

Heat Exhaustion

The symptoms of heat prostration and collapse are weakness and dizziness, headache and faintness. The skin becomes cold and clammy and grey in appearance. The pupils of the eyes are dilated, temperatures below normal.

First-Aid. Primarily rest in an air-conditioned or cool room, but if the athlete does not recover he may need medical aid.

Heat Stroke

The symptoms are almost the opposite of heat exhaustion. The temperature can be very high and the skin hot and dry. The condition is caused by a breakdown in the sweating mechanism. This can be serious.

First-Aid. The body must be cooled immediately with cold wet towels applied to the whole skin area. An ice bath could be used. The athlete's temperature must be lowered as heat stroke can be a killer if the temperature is not reduced.

Effects of Cold Weather

If a warm track suit is not kept on until just before an event, or the warm-up is insufficient to get the muscles into good working order, damage to muscles is extremely likely.

Equestrian Sports: Flat Racing, Steeplechase, Hurdles, Hunting, Eventing, Show Jumping, Polo

Equestrian injuries in flat racing, steeplechase, hurdles, hunting, eventing, show jumping and so on are similar and only differ in possible frequency and severity. In falling, the rider can best prevent serious injury by falling *away* from the horse, releasing the reins at once so as to effect a clean separation. If this is not possible the horse, in falling, may roll on top of his rider. The rider can also be badly kicked not only by his own horse but by those jumping behind him. If the skull is kicked this can be serious and would probably cause concussion and possibly brain damage. Injuries to the chest, ribs, damage to the chest wall and even to the underlying lungs can occur. Fractures of the spine (vertebrae) are fairly common and can be serious, causing possible paralysis of the limbs and even death. *First-Aid* in any such serious injuries should not be given by any inexperienced person as he might do more harm than good. In most equestrian sports of this type an ambulance is in the neighbourhood to convey the injured rider to hospital.

FRACTURED COLLAR BONE
By far the most frequent injury is a fractured collar bone (clavicle).
First-Aid. The arm and shoulder must be carefully immobilised with a temporary sling with as little movement as possible.

FLAT RACING INJURIES
An injury specific to flat racing is caused by the horse being nudged out of line and getting his legs crossed. If the jockey is pressed right up against the rails so that he is squashed between the horse and railing he may get contusion and bruising or a broken bone in the lower leg.
First-Aid. Since an ambulance will be readily available at a race course, first-aid can be left to the qualified ambulance attendants.

POLO INJURIES
As well as the injuries that can occur in any equestrian sport there are those which apply specifically to polo. Most of these derive from the use of the stick and the ball. Direct hits from either may cause *severe bruising and contusions* of the tissues. Severe bruising can also be caused when a player, in fighting to play the ball, crosses in front of his opponent. In falling, the players may be kicked either by their own or their opponents' ponies.
First-Aid. Ice compresses will lessen the pain temporarily. Any further treatment depends on how severe the bruising is.

If *spinal injuries* are suspected great care must be taken in moving the patient off the field; in fact it would be best if he were not moved at all but as he is likely to be injured on the field of play he must be transported to safety.

First-Aid. The safest way to administer first-aid without disturbing the patient is by the use of the 'Australian stretcher' described in Chapter 2. As the supports are plastic he can be X-rayed on the stretcher. This is a comparatively new invention but one which should be available where spinal damage is likely to occur. If an ordinary stretcher, or a makeshift stretcher such as a door or a gate is used, at least four people should help to move the injured player on to it so that he is kept completely immobilised. With possible severe spinal injuries there is always the danger of further injury to the spinal cord with the possibility of paralysis.

Polo places a great *strain on the arm* carrying the polo stick and this can take the form of strains on the outer side of the forearm (the extensor supinator group as in 'tennis elbow') or of the inner muscles of the forearm (the flexor pronator group as in 'golfer's elbow').

First-Aid. In either case the arm must be rested in a sling. If a universal sling is not available a scarf or other temporary sling should be used. Medical attention must be sought as the whole arm must be treated.

Since the polo stick is either held in the hand and steadied by a loop which passes over the thumb, or else with the loop passed around the wrist, injuries can result from the stick being forced out of the player's hand by his opponent. In the first case the *thumb joint may be strained, sprained, dislocated or subluxed.* In the second the *wrist can be dislocated* and possibly also the *shoulder.*

First-Aid. Since it is impossible to tell exactly how severe the damage is without proper diagnostic tools including X-ray, immobilisation of the part, plus cold or ice compresses to help relieve pain, is all that can be carried out on the scene.

Field Sports:
Baseball, Basketball, Cricket, Hockey, Hurling, Lacrosse

SCRAPED SKIN (ABRASIONS)

Common to most of these sports. 'Strawberries' – sometimes called 'mat burns' – affect **baseball** players on hips, buttocks and the back of the thighs when sliding into base. In **basketball** falling or skidding on the hardwood floor results in scraped knees or elbows.

First-Aid. In all cases the wound should immediately be cleansed with soap and water and a mild disinfectant applied with a sterile dry dressing to protect the damaged surface from infection. If there is any dirt in the wound likely to cause inflammation or abscessing it must be treated by a doctor.

DIRECT BLOWS

In sports where a hard ball is used varying degrees of injury to the face and head or other parts of the body can occur. Heads can also clash. In **basketball** an occasional concussion has resulted from heads meeting below the basket. In **cricket** a batsman can receive hits on various parts of the body from the bowler and he, too, may be concussed by a blow to the head. In **hockey** uneven ground can cause the ball to rise at an awkward angle when two players go for it simultaneously. Concussion here is rare but a black eye is common. In **hurling**, a wild Irish form of hockey, there is danger from both ball and stick as sticks can be clashed in the air as well as on the ground and heads are likely to be hit. A direct hit from a ball, which can travel distances of seventy-five yards in the air, can produce a nasty bump. In **lacrosse** goalies risk concussion but are more likely to get loosened front teeth or a bloody nose.

First-Aid. All cases of suspected *concussion* must be treated very seriously and the player must never return to the game even if he appears to have recovered but should immediately be seen by a doctor.

Ice-packs will reduce the painful swelling of *bruising* on the face, around the eye or on the forehead. It is also the best treatment for *bloody noses.* As well as an ice-pack on the nose, one can be placed on the back of the neck and the bleeding nostril packed with gauze or cotton wool. Bruises on other parts of the body do not usually require the player to come off the field unless the skin is broken, in which case he should stop play long enough for the wound to be cleaned and dressed with sterile gauze and adhesive tape, after which he can usually return to the game.

KNEE INJURIES

These occur in **baseball**, **basketball** and **hockey** and, to a lesser extent, in other field sports. Ligaments may be torn as the result of many violent twisting movements and sudden stops. Another type of knee injury can be caused by either stick or ball, resulting in internal bleeding into the joint. *First-Aid.* Protection of the knee joint with strapping may afford some degree of stability in the case of a torn ligament but the player must stop play and if the tear is severe it may need surgical supervision. In the case of a hard blow causing internal bleeding into the joint (haemarthrosis) aspiration by a surgeon will be required and an elastic felt pad (an arthropad) applied.

FINGER AND HAND INJURIES
These are frequent in **baseball**, **basketball**, **cricket**, **hockey** and **lacrosse**, though not always for the same reason. So-called 'baseball finger' results from catching the ball on the extended fingers. If the tip of the finger is hit by the ball subluxations and dislocations may occur. In **basketball** so-called 'jammed finger' can have a similar result, or it may cause a fracture. Wicketkeepers in **cricket** have suffered fractures of nearly every bone in the hands and fingers. Right-handed batsmen facing fast bowling often develop a thickening of the bone of the right index finger due to constant jarring; left-handers get this on their left index finger. The index finger becomes painful and this is due to a fibrous or bony thickening of the surface of the bone (the periosteum).
First-Aid. For fractured fingers this consists of binding the injured finger to the next with full hyperextension. When more than one finger is injured and there is swelling and pain the player must come off the field and receive medical attention. For fibrous or bony thickening rest and protection is essential.

HITS ON THE SHIN
These can occur from either stick or ball and are very painful.
First-Aid. Ice packs can relieve the pain. Bandaging is only necessary if the wound is open. Shin bruises take a long time to heal but will not prevent a keen player from returning to his sport.

CHARLEYHORSE (LOCALISED INTRAMUSCULAR TEAR)
May have several causes: a direct hit from a ball or stick, or an overload of

the muscles from fatigue, or by the sudden application of stress to a muscle-tendo-bone unit which exceeds its tolerance. The muscles in front of the thigh (quadriceps) are sometimes involved. Muscle fibres are torn and bruising and blood formation (haematoma) result.

First-Aid. Ice-packs may reduce pain followed by the late Doctor Austin Moore's SUELMEX treatment: Support, Elevation, Massage and Exercise.

STRAIN OR TEAR OF THIGH OR CALF
These result, in **baseball**, from a quick run between bases and in **cricket** between wickets.

Fighting Sports: Boxing, Fencing

BOXING
Dr J. L. Blonstein, one of the world's foremost medical boxing experts, has said that what is most surprising about boxing injuries is that there are far fewer of them than would be expected, fewer than in any kind of football, for instance. However, since a good many boxing injuries are to the face they probably show more.

Nosebleed
This is certainly the most frequent.

First-Aid. An ice pack held over the nose, packing the nostrils with strips of gauze (though this can force the blood into the mouth which may cause vomiting) or a roll of gauze packed between the upper teeth and lip may, by exerting pressure, stop the bleeding.

Cauliflower Ears
These are caused more by half-evading a blow, resulting in constant friction and small haemorrhaging, than by direct blows. The small haematomas gradually organise into fibrous tissue which in time causes deformity.

First-Aid. Initially ice packs may disperse the haematomas lessening their chance of organising.

Eyes
Damage to the skin around the eyes is common. This can be in the form of cuts or bruises which may initially be caused by the opponent's head but also by punches. The eye itself is rarely damaged, being protected by the surrounding bones.

First-Aid. Lacerated eyelids usually bleed profusely and the bleeding should be controlled with a pressure dressing soaked in an astringent, using direct hand pressure – provided there is no damage to the eye itself. The affected area should then be covered with a loose dressing. Lacerations below the eye do not bleed so much but should be treated with a lightly applied sterile dressing as soon as the boxer comes out of the ring.

Knuckles and Hands
Despite bandages worn under the gloves, hands are frequently injured. Contusions of the soft tissue at the back of the hands can happen, knuckles can be bruised or cut and there may be sprains or fractures of the finger bones (metacarpal). The famous boxer Henry Cooper recommends cotton bandages held together with zinc oxide strapping rather than crepe. Only by minute attention to the preparation of the bandage and tape, he says, can some of these injuries be forestalled.

First-Aid. If one finger is broken it can be taped to the adjacent finger. If more than one they must be treated by a doctor.

Contrast bathing for treating bruised hands is better than ice-packs right from the beginning. The heat soaks diffuse the bruising to the surrounding tissues by dilating the tissues, and the contrasting cold water constricts the vessels and thereby creates an alternating action on the blood vessels which makes for quick absorption of the traumatic swelling. Some authorities think that this is controversial because the hot compresses could allow the continuation of bleeding. In fact, this very rarely happens.

Elbows
Constant jarring of the elbows, particularly the right-handed boxer's left

elbow (right elbow in a southpaw) initially causes jarring of the bones with pain and in time loose bodies and eventually osteoarthritis due to cartilage injury may appear in the elbow joint.

First-Aid. Contrast bathing as above.

Bruised Ribs
Caused by body punching.

First-Aid. Some doctors advocate the use of an enzyme such as varidase to cut down on the effects of bruising. Homoeopathic doctors recommend arnica.

FENCING

Muscle Strains or Pulls
Pulled muscles or strained back are often caused by the reversal of force. Strains of the elbow are also common, causing pain when certain movements are checked, as in the completion of 'parry seconde'. Strains or sprains of the back at waist-level due to twisting movements can sometimes lead to disc trouble. Strains of the shoulder joint are common and sometimes result in a lesion of the shoulder muscle (supraspinatous syndrome).

First-Aid. Strains or sprains need rest from the sport and, in the case of upper limbs, rest in a sling. Hot and cold contrast baths or compresses are useful. If pain persists, or if the sprain is severe, medical attention must be sought.

Penetration Injuries
With the use of protective clothing and epée points, this type of injury is rare. If the point of the weapon is accidentally broken off, or if it snaps lower on the epée, the remaining point is much sharper than the normally safe point. Even here the broken weapon is quickly withdrawn, although the fencer's reflexes may not be quick enough to stop his forward lunge in time, and the protective clothing may have become worn or the mask rusted. This is, fortunately, unlikely: Olympic epée finalist and surgeon, R. Porritt, reports only two fatal accidents and these were far apart – one in 1937 and the other in 1951. Both these fatalities were caused by a weak

spot in the protective clothing over the inner armpit and in both cases lungs were pierced. They resulted in a further reconsideration of the defensive rules.

Lesser degrees of injury could be lacerations of the neck or arms and there is always the possibility in such cases of an artery being pierced, especially in the neck.

First-Aid. Where an artery has been pierced there will be spurts of blood at the same speed as the beats of the heart and manual pressure will have to be applied to stop the bleeding. Pressure should be applied both above and below the point of bleeding.

Impact Injuries
A fencer can trip and fall, be knocked down by the opponent or driven back to bump against the wall of the salle. On occasion an epée can produce a long weal similar to a blow from a cane or a whip.

First-Aid For abrasions or weals, cleanse with a mild disinfectant and apply a sterile covering to broken skin area.

Fractures of Little Finger
Little fingers can be broken by contact with the opponent's epée.

First-Aid. Splint the little finger to the ring finger by taping them together.

Football: Association, Australian, Gaelic, Rugby League, Rugby Union

CUTS, CONTUSIONS AND BRUISES
In all forms of football direct injuries can consist of every kind of bump, bruise, kick or even scratch. In Australian rules almost anything goes except, fortunately, hitting or kicking below the belt or above the shoulder. In spite of this, severe bruising may also appear on the thighs. Knee and ankle injuries caused by kicks are common in soccer. In Gaelic football, since body charges are allowed as well as shoulder punching,

there may be a good deal of bruising. The rules allow the ball to be fisted and a player can often fist an opponent instead of the ball. If this blow lands in the eye it is likely to cause a black eye, though permanent damage is usually prevented by bony protection surrounding the eye.

In rugby, league and union, cuts, especially of the eyebrow, and tears of the ear can result from heads colliding in the ruck, the scrum or the line-out.

First-Aid can usually be applied on the field with bucket and sponge and Band-aid, sterile packs and Elastoplast unless the cut is so deep that it will need stitching, in which case the player must come off the field. By Australian rules first-aid is performed on the field without halting the game; the teams have several trainers who work with the game going on around these injured players. If a player is hurt seriously enough to retire, a substitute takes his place and he may not return during the course of that game.

SPRAINS AND STRAINS

Strains, sprains and pulled muscles usually happen at the beginning of the game when the player is cold, or at the end when he is tired and actions may be carelessly performed.

In soccer, sprains of ankles and knees are most frequent and this is also true of Australian rules. In Gaelic football ankles also suffer as a result of high jumping to catch the ball which is a feature of the game. This happens when the player lands on an unbalanced ankle and ricks over. In rugger, shoulder and neck injuries are more usual because of the pressures and strains of the scrum; however, ankles, knees, hamstrings and calf muscles are often affected. In the ankle the outside (lateral) side of the joint is usually involved whereas it is the inner side of the knee which is affected by twisting falls or by another player hitting or falling on the outer side of the knee of his opponent.

First-Aid. If the degree of the injury is mild a supportive bandage may allow the player to return to the game. If it is more severe he must come off the field and get medical aid.

DISLOCATIONS AND SUBLUXATIONS

In any form of football, falls on the outstretched hands may result in dislocations or subluxations of the elbow, shoulder or collarbone (clavicle). Falls on the shoulder, as may easily happen in rugger, have a similar result. In rugger, dislocated bones of the fingers are caused by a player handling the ball just as another decides to kick it. In Gaelic football players often injure their fingers in catching the ball.

First-Aid. Finger dislocations can usually be treated on the field but the player may suffer intense pain if the bone is pressing on a nerve and reduction on the field impossible. However, a dislocation is always best reduced immediately if this can be done. The bones should be pulled apart so as to stretch the joint capsule. Twisting or pressure, with the bony ends in alignment, will cause the displaced end of the distal bone to fall into place. The player may be able to do this himself but in the case of a major joint reduction it is better left to a doctor as there may be complications.

FRACTURES

Fractures may happen in any kind of football. Falls on the wrist can cause a break of three bones (radius, ulna and scaphoid). Falls on the hands often cause a collarbone (clavicle) to snap.

If one player falls across another player's leg, either or both bones (fibula and tibia) may be broken. A broken finger, usually the index, can be caused by catching the ball incorrectly.

First-Aid. Except for a finger, which can be splintered to an adjacent finger, a fracture victim should receive medical attention at the earliest possible moment. Meanwhile, the patient should be made as comfortable as possible and some sort of temporary splint used (a rolled newspaper, a stick or, in the case of the leg, the adjacent leg) in order to prevent aggravation of the break by movement. If the wound is open (compound) a sterile dressing should be placed on the wound: if necessary the adjacent clothing should be gently cut away.

TEARS OF MUSCLES OR TENDONS

Tears of calf muscles, of the knee cartilage and of the tendons at the back of the ankles (tendo-Achilles) are sometimes caused by the player pivoting suddenly, or by any twisting, extension or flexion movements.

E

First-Aid. Cold compresses to help reduce pain and swelling; rest and elevation.

NOSEBLEEDS
Common to any kind of football.

First-Aid. The flow can sometimes be arrested by the sponge-and-bucket man. If not, the player must come off the field and apply ice and a cottonwool plug for the nostril. Ice at the back of the neck sometimes helps.

CONCUSSION
Brain concussion of any severity should have complete rest, avoiding bright lights, reading or television. The player must not return to the game until all symptoms have been removed for at least a month.

PROTECTIVE CLOTHING
In American football many injuries are caused by the clothing worn for protection. Three out of four of the injuries caused by this hazardous clothing are severe enough to keep the player out of the sport for four or more days.

The helmet is probably the most lethal since players use it for 'spearing', driving it into various part of the opponent's anatomy. This can cause internal injuries or deep bruising (haematoma). In addition, the aggressor himself may damage the vertebrae in his own neck as a result of compression. Another cause of extensive injuries of the neck comes from a certain form of illegal tackling when a player grabs his opponent's face-guard and uses it to 'wrench his head off' by pulling it violently, the back part of the helmet acting as a fulcrum on the back part of the neck (cervical spine).

Cleated shoes cause ankle and knee strains. When the foot is planted and the player tackled from the outer side the inner ligaments of the knee are subject to tearing especially if he is swerving at the time. This tends to happen if his foot is facing in one direction and his body is twisted to go in another to avoid being tackled. Leg cartilages (menisci) can also receive rotation injuries.

66

First-Aid. Many American football clubs use a jet of hot water producing a whirlpool called a 'de Cussie' at first, followed by ice-packs and support.

Mechanical Sports: Cycle Racing, Motor Cycle Racing, Motor Racing

CYCLE RACING

The loneliness of long-distance cycling is ensured by competitors starting at intervals of some minutes, their time recorded on stop watches, so that there is no visible competitor to beat. Long distances, long hours – not surprising, perhaps, that the racing cyclist took to pep pills (amphetamines). It was not until a top rider died from the effect of the drug in 1967 that much more stringent rules were instituted and daily tests made.

Vascular Disorders

The constant pressure on a cyclist's legs can cause *varicose veins*. These are veins that have lost their elasticity; they have a bluish, knotted, tortuous appearance. The veins are dilated by the inability of the weakened venous walls to withstand the pressure of the blood in their veins, in which case the valves which normally prevent this fail to function properly and a reversal of blood in the vein may occur.

First-Aid. Any cyclist with a tendency to varicose veins should wear firm support stockings and elevate his legs when at rest. If a vein bursts, the bleeding must be stopped by direct pressure or compression both above and below the injury and the leg elevated. Later a doctor should be consulted who could prescribe injections of substances which cause the vein to harden and ultimately become less painful. If these do not work, operation may be necessary.

Another vascular disturbance to which cyclists are prone – due to pressure of the blood vessels of the lower part of the leg – is *clotting of the blood in the veins* (thrombophlebitis). This is caused by a condition of congestion which can put the leg muscles (anterior tibial) at risk. The loss of the blood supply may cause death of the tissues (necrosis).

First-Aid. Elevation of the leg with the application of ice compresses. Immediate removal to hospital as an operation may be urgently needed to save the muscles of the lower leg.

MOTOR CYCLE RACING
Almost any kind of injury can result from a spill.

Strains and Sprains
In speedway, dragging the left foot may result in strains or sprains on the inside of the ankle or knee as a result of jarring the foot on the rough surface.

First-Aid. Hot and cold compresses will help relieve pain and swelling. The injured part should then be bound with a stretch bandage fastened firmly but not so tight as to interfere with the circulation.

Bruises and Abrasions
Bruises and abrasions, with the addition of cinder burns which may cause an open contaminated wound, possibly haemorrhaging, often happen.

First-Aid. The object will be to control bleeding as far as possible. It is better not to attempt to remove cinders or dirt from the wound as this may cause further haemorrhaging. Bleeding can be controlled with a dressing held by the hand or by a pressure bandage but, if the wound is contaminated, it is essential to get the rider to a medical centre where it can be expertly cleaned.

Fractures
Fractures are most likely to occur in an arm or a leg.

First-Aid. Clothing should be cut away and the limb immobilised by some sort of splint. If the fracture has caused an open wound (compound fracture) great care must be taken to avoid further infection.

MOTOR RACING
Accidents, when they hapen, are usually serious. In a crash a driver may

68

be trapped or the car may catch fire before he has been able to get out.

Burns

The driver may receive severe burns on any part of his body or face. The respiratory tract can also suffer heat damage with the result that breathing becomes difficult.

Burns cause shock, due both to fluid loss and extreme pain. The seriousness of the burn depends on how much of the body has been affected, as well as the degree of the burns. A first-degree burn is not very serious as it affects only the superficial layer of the skin with reddening. A second-degree burn damages a deeper level and is shown by blistering. It is serious if burns cover more than thirty per cent of the body area. A third-degree burn is the most serious: it goes to the full depth of the skin and sometimes destroys the sensory nerves (and with these the sensation of pain).

Even third-degree burns may be 'minor' if they cover only two per cent of the body surface and exclude face, hands and feet. They are 'moderate' if they cover from two to ten per cent without involving face, hands or feet. They are 'severe', probably critical, if more than ten per cent of the body surface is burned with the face, hands, feet and respiratory tract involved.

First-Aid. Grease or oil of any sort should never be used for burns. Apply local treatment using cold wet applications for relief of pain. Cover the burned area with a sterile dressing or a clean sheet. If the victim is finding it difficult to breathe try to establish an open airway or, if available, use an oxygen-adding first-aid device. Prevent the loss of heat by putting blankets gently over the victim but do not add heat. As he is probably in shock, do not give any liquids, particularly alcoholic stimulants. The most urgent efforts should be made to get the victim to medical attention, preferably to a hospital with a burns unit.

Concussion

This is by far the most frequent injury, despite crash helmets. It may not always be immediately obvious: the driver who has been thrown clear often gets up and declares he is uninjured, and drivers have been known to run down a track for as much as a hundred yards before collapsing unconscious, suffering from delayed reaction.

First-Aid. A driver who is so badly hurt that he is rendered unconscious should be covered with a rug and, if is avoidable, not moved until the ambulance arrives. If he must be moved to get him out of the way of other motor cars, it should be to the nearest verge and with the greatest possible care as the spinal cord could be damaged. Make sure that he is breathing properly and examine eyes, nose, ears and mouth for possible haemorrhaging.

If a driver has been involved in an accident, even if he is not apparently injured, he should not drive for at least a week as there is always the danger of delayed shock. In a fast race this could cause him to become involved in a further accident.

Racquet Sports: Tennis, Squash, Badminton, Table Tennis, Pelota

Certain injuries are common to all sports played with a racquet.

TWISTING INJURIES

These are becoming increasingly frequent. Many courts now used are made of synthetic grass which gives a good grip and enables the player to accelerate quickly. Unfortunately, this has some disadvantages. For one thing it triples the danger of injuries which are due to sudden stops and starts. In polychloride surfaces such as Initurf or Supreme Turf (which is polyvinyl), with a canvas backing laid over a packed surface, quick stops and turns causing foot and knee injuries are inevitable.

Again, heat can build up from a relatively impervious surface rising to 110° F on artificial grass while the surrounding air may be under 80° F. The common practice of wetting down the surface may or may not aid the condition though it does somewhat decrease the friction coefficient which causes the twisting injuries, says New York orthopaedic surgeon Arthur Bernhang.

First-Aid. If the condition is a strained ankle and is not too bad, and if the match is important, put a firm stretch bandage round the ankle. If it is painful to put the foot to the ground, the player must come off and treatment must be instigated.

TENNIS ELBOW

In all sports played with a racquet so-called 'tennis elbow' is frequent. It can start with a feeling of fatigue after half-an-hour's practice or one or two

70

sets. The grip weakens and, possibly after a mis-hit shot, pain begins, and may get progressively worse, on the outside of the elbow. The actual injury is a strain or partial tear at the origin of some of the muscle fibres on the outer side of the elbow. As a result, this releases inflammatory exudations which cause pain and swelling.

First-Aid. At the first sign of arm fatigue the arm should be rested in a sling, even if it means cutting out potentially profitable tournaments; it will save time in the long run. Ice-packs can be used to lessen pain. A doctor may recommend physiotherapy.

Often involved with tennis elbow is the tendon in front of the shoulder as the biceps is the principle fixor of the elbow and rotator of the forearm in the backhand action.

CALF MUSCLE TEARS AND STRAINS

These may be caused by excessive stretching and the muscle may be only partially torn. The first sign is when the player feels as if he had received a sharp blow on the back of the upper calf muscles. The exact point of pain reveals which muscle is involved and the point of tear.

First-Aid. With more than a very mild degree of pain, the player should at once stop playing to avoid further tears or even rupture. Ice-packs will help relieve pain and the leg should be bandaged and elevated.

BRUISING

A **squash** player could be bruised by hitting the walls of the court.

First-Aid. A small bruise requires no special attention but if there is swelling and bleeding under the skin, ice-packs or cold compresses will help reduce the swelling; padding and a soft roller bandage for pressure may bring relief. If the bruise is large and contains blood and serum, the doctor or surgeon will probably recommend aspirating the products of the bruise (haematoma) through a large bore needle under a local anaesthetic, as if they are allowed to remain various complications, such as painful thickenings, could result.

ABRASION

If a player falls hard on the court he may cause an abrasion.

First-Aid. This must be treated seriously, especially if considerable skin surface has been lost, even though there is very little bleeding and the wound is shallow, as there is always the possibility of infection. The wound should be bathed with a mild disinfectant and covered with sterile gauze. Unless the wound becomes inflamed through sepsis, it will probably not need further medical attention.

EYE INJURIES

Pelota, sometimes known as **jai alai**, can be hazardous if the player receives a direct hit from the hard ball travelling at speed. If the player is hard hit over the eye, a bad bruise or a black eye is usually the extent of the damage, due to the bony protection round the eye. But occasionally the eyelid can be lacerated.

First-Aid. Soft tissue injuries to the eyelid may appear more serious than they are but, as long as the eyeball itself is unharmed, vision will not be affected. Since these wounds often bleed profusely the first step is to control this by direct hand pressure with a sterile dressing. However, if the eyeball itself is damaged – lacerated – pressure should not be used. A protective dressing without pressure should be applied, and the person should be taken to hospital immediately.

Solo Sports: Game Shooting, Golf

GAME SHOOTING

Gun-Shot Wounds

Game shooting is only really dangerous if the fellow guns rather than the game get shot and this can happen, though more often in fiction than in fact. Shooting accidents are almost always attributable to carelessness or ignorance. Not everybody who buys a licence for a shotgun (or buys a shotgun without a licence) is a responsible person. In the hands of one who is inexperienced a shotgun is more dangerous than a rifle.

Internal bleeding almost always results from a penetration wound of the chest, the extent depending on the depth and severity of the injury. Air may also enter the chest cavity.

First-Aid. Where the wound is in the leg or arm, and there is bleeding from a vein (venous haemorrhage), it can usually be controlled by direct pressure applied to the wound by means of a thick sterile gauze. Bleeding from the artery (arterial haemorrhage) in the arm or leg can be controlled by the application of pressure points. These pressure points can be found at any point where an artery passes over a bony prominence so that it can be felt. Bleeding from a severed artery causes blood to spurt at each heart beat.

In a lesser wound, infection may be the danger and it is important that it should be properly treated at once, which means that those responsible for the shoot should see that a first-aid kit is available.

Although sportsmen do not normally anticipate getting shot it is advisable to have toxoid or anti-tetanus injections beforehand.

Injuries from Recoil

When a gun is fired, though the forward force propels the shot towards the target, the backward force produces a backward kick or recoil. The main force of this recoil is taken by the shoulder against which the stock is resting, although the arm may reduce the strength of the kickback. This can, at times, produce an injury to the shoulder or clavicle, especially if they have been weakened by previous injury, possibly at another sport. *First-Aid.* The sport should be discontinued and the arm rested in a universal sling, if available, or with a temporary sling made from a scarf.

Shoulder injury is usually caused by an ill-fitting stock or an incorrect mounting; before the sport is taken up again after the injury has healed, the fault in the shotgun should be corrected by a gunsmith or there will be a recurrence. Bruising of the cheek can be prevented by the fitting of a suitable pad to the stock.

Gun Headache

This can be another result of recoil, also easier to prevent than to cure. It may be a severe migrainous headache, produced by the repeated jarring or jolting of the head by recoil, which should be kept within the tolerance of the sportsman. If he has a tendency to osteoarthritis of the top of the spine, even the slightest recoil may cause a headache. *First-Aid.* A painkiller, such as aspirin, is the obvious first-aid. If the continuation of the sport without pain is the object, a good gunsmith should again be called in. The length and weight of the gun and the possibility of using a lighter load cartridge should be discussed.

Finger Fractures

These can be caused by a stock that is not the correct length as well as by recoil – and here again a gunsmith should be consulted.

First-Aid. Broken fingers should be splinted. If only one finger is broken, the adjacent finger can be used. If more than one is broken, medical attention is advisable but a pencil or thin stick could be used as a temporary measure.

GOLF

Strains and Sprains

Since in one golf stroke or another, most muscles in the body are used, strains of all sorts are possible and particularly, of course, twisting strains of the back, hip, knees and shoulders.

Strains of the low back muscles are most common, with those of the ribs and neck coming second and third. Stiff areas in the spine are predisposing factors, possibly caused by degenerative changes since it is a game in which many older people take part. Former injuries may be reactivated or strains may occur where a movable joint adjoins a stiff one.

Strains of the elbow are frequent, 'golfers' elbow' being as common as 'tennis elbow'. The strain, however, is on the opposite side of the elbow, and on the right arm (except in a left-handed player). The pain is on the inner side of the elbow and is caused by the over-use of the surrounding muscles brought about by the swing-through action of the arm combined with a too-tight grip by the hands.

So-called 'tennis elbow' can also plague a golfer with the pain being over the outer side of the elbow in a right-handed golfer and often radiating down the back of the forearm. This is due to repeated irritation of the nerve of the forearm.

Shoulder strains to right-handed golfers frequently occur as a result of pinching inflamed structures on the outer side of the left shoulder (supraspinatous syndrome) caused by the follow-through.

Inflammation of the tendon in the front of the shoulder (tenosynovitis) can be associated with the strain of the forearm due to the over-use of this tendon in working the elbow joint. (The tendon of the long head of biceps is the main flexor and supinator of the elbow joint.)

Strains or sprains to the inner side of the knee in older golfers are

74

common due to walking on rough ground with the addition of strain placed on the inner ligaments and muscles in making the shot.

Various foot strains can be due to the same uneven walking.

First-Aid. For each of these injuries the treatment is similar. Contrast baths – first with very hot water, then with ice cold and ending with hot; gentle massage of the area, kaolin poultices and exercises without strain. Another form of first-aid goes by the letters ICE – which stand for Ice, Compression and Exercise. It is unlikely that first-aid will remove the more serious symptoms which must be treated by a specialist and physiotherapist.

An electric cart, while it may save certain strains, is no absolute guarantee of safety since carts have been known to turn over on rough ground, sometimes causing complicated fractures of the thigh bone (femur). However, this is much less likely to happen than a back strain of varying intensity caused by a player, with an osteoarthritic tendency, having to carry his own bag.

Water Sports: Swimming, Diving, Water Polo, Snorkeling, Scuba Diving, Water Skiing, Surfing, Rowing, Canoeing, Yachting

In all water sports there is always the danger of drowning. First-aid and a knowledge of resuscitation may minimise the risk.

METHODS OF RESUSCITATION

The Sylvester Method
The victim is placed on his back. The first-aider sits at his head, grasps his arms and slowly draws them up to approximately a 90° angle. He then sharply moves the arms back to the victim's sides. The arms should be pressed against the chest. Repeat until breathing is restored.

Mouth-to-Mouth Resuscitation

The first-aider should first clear the victim's nose and throat of any obstruction such as false teeth, nose plugs, etc. Next take his head and place it in full backward extension. Open the mouth, pinch the nose and breathe into the victim's mouth. Every ten seconds release the mouth, listen for expelled air, breathe in and repeat until breathing is restored.

Mouth-to-Nose Resuscitation

This is only used when, for one reason or another, mouth-to-mouth is not possible. It is similar except that the victim's mouth is kept closed and the first-aider breathes or blows into the nose.

ASPHYXIA

The stoppage of breathing is sometimes the result of a diving accident and here again the best first-aid treatment is mouth-to-mouth or mouth-to-nose. The head and neck position in relation to the body is of first importance. The head must be tilted well back with the front of the neck stretched.

If the heart has also stopped, a second helper should kneel, place the heel of his right hand on the centre of the victim's chest, then, with his left hand on his right, press downward, compressing the rib cage about an inch. The release of pressure should be sudden and the whole procedure carried out at a rate of sixty to eighty times a minute. Meanwhile, the mouth-to-mouth or mouth-to-nose is continued by the first helper.

Clearly medical assistance must be obtained as soon as possible but if there is only one rescuer this may not be possible. If it is, then a cardio-pulmonary machine may become available.

INJURIES IN SWIMMING

Strains

In breast stroke a powerful and somewhat unnatural thrust of both legs with full extension of the hips, knees and ankles may cause a strain or even a tear of the hip (adductor) muscles and occasionally of the knee joint ligament but such tears do not normally happen in non-competitive

76

swimming. They can occur if the racing swimmer is under par and puts a violent effort into the closing strokes of the race.

First-Aid. Support and protection of the injured limb should be provided with towelling or rolled newspaper.

Sprains of the Wrist and Injured Fingers

These are frequent in racing turns where too violent contact with the end of the bath occurs. Subluxation or dislocation may also occur.

First-Aid. Support of a sprained wrist can be provided with a towel sling. Broken, dislocated or subluxed fingers will need qualified assistance to reduce or splint.

'Swimmer's Shoulder'

With the crawl, 'swimmer's shoulder' can be caused by the type of arm recovery used in the stroke. When the arm is brought up from the side of the thigh the shoulder is pushed upward as the hand is lifted from the water, rotated until the arm with the elbow extended goes ahead of the swimmer ready to start the next downstroke. This gives a complete rotation of the shoulder, placing considerable strain on the shoulder blade which may cause strain of the muscles or sprain of the joint itself.

First-Aid consists of putting the arm in an improvised towel sling. Treatment from the medical team will include physiotherapy, rest and rehabilitation.

Blast Injury (Diving)

An inexpert diver can land too flat which may cause him to spit blood due to injury to the lungs. If he tackles the high board before he is sufficiently experienced, falling flat on his stomach, he may get a blast injury. Severe shock, bruising of the chest wall and possible nosebleed may result.

First-Aid. The patient should lie absolutely flat unless nosebleed causes blood to choke him, in which case lying on the side with the nostrils plugged with cottonwool is the best procedure.

Head and Neck Injuries (Diving)

A diver has been known to hit his head on the diving board after an incorrectly performed spin or twist and get concussed. Diving into a too-shallow garden pool and hitting his head on the bottom may also cause concussion or even a broken neck. In either case he will probably come to the surface face downwards and unless he is retrieved immediately will certainly drown. Unless the neck is broken below the sixth vertebra the accident may be fatal – below the sixth he can survive with proper handling in getting him out of the water. With improper handling, he may be paralysed or may still die, especially if the broken neck had not up till then caused spinal-cord damage.

First-Aid. Great care must be exercised in getting the victim out of the water to see that his head does not flop backward or bend forward or bend or twist to either side. If he is lying face downward, someone must keep the head rigid while others carefully turn him over. Then a board must be placed under him and he must be lifted out of the water very carefully, his head protected from any movement. An ironing board, surfboard, door or backboard could be used in the emergency. Start mouth-to-mouth ventilation if necessary. He should be lifted into an ambulance without being moved from the board.

Fungus Infection

A minor hazard of swimming pools is the possibility of picking up a fungus infection. The most likely type is the one commonly called athlete's foot which is both infectious and water borne and is rampant around the damp edges of swimming pools and public showers.

First-Aid is less important than prevention because, once acquired, a fungus infection is hard to cure and, even if the patient is apparently symptom-free, often reappears. The most effective deterrent is a skin kept in a condition which is alien to fungi. Dry feet thoroughly when emerging from the water and use an anti-fungoid powder each time between the toes and in socks or shoes.

Foot Injuries

Hazards common to ocean swimming are injuries to the feet caused by sharp shells, broken glass, stings or bites from marine life, coral burns and barbs from sea urchins.

Cuts

First-Aid. Cuts must be carefully treated to avoid sepsis. Using seawater, rinse the sand or grit from the wound. If nothing is embedded in the sole of the foot, clean carefully with a mild antiseptic and warm water as soon as possible and apply a sterile dressing or large Band-aid. A protective

78

stretch bandage may be placed over the dressing. If bits of shell or glass have become embedded, do not remove as this may cause bleeding; they will have to be taken out by minor surgery.

Sea Urchins

Sea urchins are prevalent in shallow water on many beaches. When stepped on, they release dozens of small barbs. These are difficult to get out.

First-Aid. Each barb may have to be removed with tweezers but they may come out if meat tenderiser (which is made of papaya) is moistened to form a paste and applied to the feet. This dissolves the spines. If the tenderiser is unavailable, ammonia is sometimes successful, which is possibly why island natives soak their barbed feet in urine. Lemon juice, too, sometimes works.

Jellyfish

Jellyfish, particularly Portuguese men o' war can cause very painful stings. Lying on a beach or floating in the shallows, a Portuguese man o' war looks innocuous, a child's toy, but the sting is in the end of a long, black trailer which is poisonous long after the main body has been washed up on the beach and died. This trailer is crammed with stinging cells and it can wind itself around hand, arm, leg or neck.

First-Aid. Using plenty of wet sand, remove the trailer. As soon as possible apply ammonia, a household blue bag or methylated spirits, followed by an analgesic cream. Wherever there is the possibility of stings from sea creatures one of these remedies should always be carried in the beach bag.

Sea Wasp

In tropical waters a sting from a jellyfish known as a *sea wasp* can be dangerous as a snake bite and should be treated similarly.

First-Aid. A constricting band should be tied both above and below the injury close to, but not on, the swelling caused by the bite. It should not be tight enough to constrict the pulse below it. The wound should be sucked without any delay. Suck and spit out. No harm will come of this unless there is an open wound in the mouth. The victim should be carried to the nearest medical aid; walking may spread the poison.

SNORKELING

A particular hazard of snorkeling – unless a diving suit is worn, which is rare among snorkelers – is the possibility of coral cuts or poisoning. Scrapes and abrasions on the sharp edges of the coral are frequent. One type, fire coral, which is a mustard colour, causes blisters (contact dermatitis) which are similar to those of poison ivy. They can last an uncomfortable length of time with severe itching.

First-Aid. The worst of the symptoms – the blistering and itching – may not occur until several days after the original contact. Blisters do not always appear: sometimes there is redness and roughness accompanied by itching, or redness and itching followed by blistering in a few days. A lotion made from diluted ammonia may relieve the itching in the first instance but should be followed by one with a calamine base with antihistamine or cortisone added. Unless the area is too large, a sterile dressing should be applied as this stops scratching and starting up a secondary infection. The condition is self-limiting unless a secondary infection occurs in which case medical treatment should be sought.

SCUBA DIVING

'Bends'

Most of the dangers of scuba diving derive from the pressure to which a diver is subjected when he descends to any depth in the ocean. This extra pressure is instantly transmitted to the whole inside of his body. Oxygen, which is fundamental in atmosphere, will, at a depth of thirty feet, become a deadly poison when breathed alone; nitrogen goes into solution in the body tissues. It is this fact which makes decompression from depths of over thirty feet necessary in order that nitrogen should come out of solution slowly. If this is not done and the diver rises too quickly, the nitrogen gradually forms bubbles in the blood stream, causing the decompression sickness known as 'bends' or 'caisson disease' (a caisson is the chamber or diving-bell once used by workers in underwater bridge building). Symptoms, which may appear several hours after surfacing, are respiratory troubles and nervous upsets, extreme fatigue and considerable pain in the joints. Rates of ascent are laid down in diving to prevent this. However, some tables are better than others.

First-Aid. Immediate recompression in the pressure chamber is essential to avoid lasting damage. High pressures will reduce the size of the bubbles and force them back into the tissues. The diver should then be more slowly decompressed so that he may exhale all the excess oxygen.

Annoxia
This is caused by an inadequate supply of oxygen in the tissues, and produces pain in the chest.

First-Aid. Application of oxygen.

Oxygen Poisoning
This is the opposite of annoxia and is caused by breathing pure oxygen under pressure. Symptoms are dizziness, muscle twitching, numbness, throat irritation and possible convulsions.

First-Aid. In the case of convulsions, airway passages must be kept open and the head protected. Prevent tongue-biting by wedging something into the mouth. Loosen clothing around the neck and chest.

Nitrogen Poisoning (Narcosis)
This is caused by deep diving (120 feet or more) and produces a cross between unconsciousness and very deep sleep. It starts, however, with euphoria or 'drunkenness' which may cause the diver to take off his breathing apparatus while under water, unable, in his disoriented state, to realise his danger. For many years experiments have been tried in which nitrogen is replaced by helium in the breathing gas. While the use of helium slows down decompression time, it does, even at depths of over 500 feet, reduce the intoxication.

First-Aid. Bring to the surface. Give artificial ventilation and oxygen.

Subcutaneous Emphysema
In this condition air is forced into the tissues from the lungs. It is possible to cause this condition when machines used in artificial respiration are operated incorrectly. The symptoms are swelling of the face, neck, chest wall, abdominal wall and scrotum.

First-Aid. The patient should immediately be transported to hospital by ambulance.

Traumatic Ear Drum Rupture
This can happen as a result of pressure. Symptoms are sharp intermittent pain, dizziness, headache, ringing sounds.
First-Aid. If there is bleeding, a small piece of sterile cottonwool can be inserted in the outer ear. Do not syringe. The condition will heal without further treatment in a few weeks but further diving should be avoided.

In the following serious diving illnesses the diver must be brought instantly to the surface and treated by a doctor.

Spontaneous Pneumothorax
This is a collection of air in the pleural cavity which causes the lungs to collapse. Symptoms are spitting up of foamy, bloody sputum, shortness of breath, bluish discoloration of the lips, finger-nails and possibly also the skin. Medical treatment consists of aspirating the air from the lung by inserting a needle. This may have to be done several times.

Air Embolism
This may occur when water pressure forces air from the lungs into the blood vessels. Air in the arteries and veins can cause serious consequences; the air bubbles in the blood vessels can reach the heart and other parts of the body preventing them from receiving oxygen and other substances needed for their survival. Symptoms are mottling or itching of the skin; nausea, dizziness and vomiting, severe pain over the part of the chest where the air embolism is lodged, with difficulty in breathing, pain in other parts of the body, in muscles, joints and tendons, impeded vision.
First-Aid. Immediate recompression in the pressure chamber must be followed, when released nitrogen is forced back into the blood, by gradual decompression. Secondary medical treatment may consist of oxygen inhalation. Artificial ventilation may be started even before transportation to hospital.

Squeeze Injuries
These cause pressure build-ups in ears, sinuses, lungs or eyes, resulting in

rupture of the blood vessels in these areas. Symptoms are blood in the ears, throat and nose, deafness, lack of co-ordination and dizziness.

First-Aid. Application of oxygen (one hundred per cent if possible) and immediate transportation to medical centre.

Contra-indications to Scuba Diving*

Fatigue. No one should dive after a long air journey or a sleepless night.

Sunstroke. If the boat is to take some time to reach the diving area, care should be taken to guard against too much sun. Barrier creams, long-sleeved shirts and hats are advisable.

Seasickness. If a person becomes seasick in the boat this will not pass off underwater and seasick remedies may cause drowsiness which would be fatal.

Physical. No one should dive if suffering from any of the following: colds, infected sinuses or ears, or any other ear trouble; any weakness of the heart, coronary vessels or cardio-vascular system; or if there is a past history of tuberculosis, however long ago and apparently cured. You should not dive if you have asthma (unless with the doctor's specific permission), sinusitis, emphysema, epilepsy, diabetes (because of the danger of coma); or if you have recently had hepatitis, nephritis or cystitis, unreduced hernia, or any sort of operation. Women should not dive if pregnant or nursing children. Many divers are injured because they are not sufficiently fit to withstand cold and exhaustion.

Psychological. Fear of water or of going beneath the surface; claustrophobia; inability to meet crises, giving in to panic – all these make diving inadvisable. Add to these the presence of show-offs or daredevils who might do foolish things which would endanger the safety of other divers.

Diving without Training. Diving equipment can be bought by anyone, trained or untrained. Accidents caused by lack of training and ignorance take place every year with unnecessary deaths. Of some 26,000–28,000 amateur divers in Great Britain only 19,000 belong to recognised clubs such as the sub-aqua clubs, which provide training, both practical and theoretical, with subsequent examinations of achievement.

* I am grateful for the information on scuba diving to Mr Harry Cox of Bermuda, who, says his father, the Hon. Sir John Cox, has been deep-diving since he was seven years old.

POSSIBLE HAZARDS AND INJURIES IN WATER SKIING

Certain types of equipment and clothing can cause risk or are not advisable. Even in warm weather the wind of speed against a wet body can bring on muscle chill; a sweater should be worn. Even if it gets wet, warm air is trapped. Bikinis are not recommended. At speed they can come off if the skier falls.

In cold weather wear an overall garment such as a track suit. In even colder weather a 'wet suit' is useful. Wet suits are made of synthetic rubber which has excellent insulating properties. Water is inserted in small quantities, is warmed by the body; and the insulated rubber keeps the warmth trapped. To be comfortable, a wet suit should be worn over woollen underwear.

Beginner's Stiffness

A beginner should wear a lifebelt and should not do more than an hour's skiing the first few times as every muscle is used and the skier can be very stiff indeed the next morning.

First-Aid. A long soak in a hot bath. Seaweed bubble bath preparation helps keep the water hot.

Falls

A detachable flag or marker will give warning to other boats if the skier should fall in the water.

After a fall, the rope can do damage; a skier may be dragged by it or it can whip round and catch arms, legs or body or twist around the neck; it may cause brush burns, or deep lacerations.

First-Aid. Cold applications will help reduce pain and swelling of closed bruises. In an open wound, bleeding must be controlled by a pressure bandage. Broken or scraped skin needs sterile dressing to keep infection from the wound pending medical attention.

A fall can also cause water to be driven at pressure into the ears creating inflammation in the middle ear (otitis media). Since ear plugs may be forced into the ear by pressure, the best prevention is a well-fitting rubber bathing cap securely fastened under the chin.

Sprains, strains, joint dislocations and tears of muscles can result from falls in the water.

84

First-Aid. Support, protection and elevation of the limb until medical aid is obtained.

INJURIES SPECIFIC TO SURFING

Competitive surfing requires a very high standard of fitness and the surfer must, of course, be a first-class swimmer. The most frequent hazard in surfing is a loose surfboard. If a surfer falls off his own board, or if another surfer's board is loose, he can receive a powerful and even dangerous blow.

First-Aid. The most important thing is to get him ashore. Then treatment, according to the area and extent of the damage, must be applied. He may need resuscitation, he may be concussed, he may have broken bones or neck, any of which would need immediate medical attention if available. Immobilisation until medical help is available is the best first-aid, except in the case of near-drowning when mouth-to-mouth or mouth-to-nose should be tried.

HAZARDS AND INJURIES IN WATER POLO

Hazards. Fouls under water which the referee cannot see are the most likely to cause minor damage, mostly bruises. Kicking or striking an opponent, submerging him, attacking an opponent who is not holding the ball, penalised if seen, can all cause minor injuries.

Injuries. Though rare, subluxed or dislocated shoulders or fingers can happen.

First-Aid. It is unlikely that someone present understands the principles of snapping a dislocated shoulder joint back into place (reducing). A player can do his own finger by pulling it from the top joint and allowing it to fall back into its socket.

BOATING

Hazards and Injuries in Rowing or Sculling

Blisters on the hands and fingers are frequent at the beginning of the season, said to be caused not only by as yet unhardened skin but also by the oar being too tightly gripped instead of lightly held. These may be prevented by surgical spirit or friar's balsam (tincture of benzoin) applied to harden the skin.

First-Aid. If the skin is broken, great care must be taken to use absolutely sterile techniques. A disinfectant with sterile bandage should be used but the rower must wait until the hand is healed before rowing again; if he rows wearing a bandage of any sort it may ruck up and make matters worse.

Blisters on the heels may occur in wet weather. An Elastoplast dressing may be used during rowing as the heel does not move enough to displace it. Aids to prevention include the use of friar's balsam and a spirit to harden the skin, and then cold cream to make it pliable.

Muscular Strains are the most common of all rowing injuries; strains to shoulder, back and abdomen, usually caused by faulty techniques. These can be prevented if the forward movement is taken as a swing from the hips and not as a forward reach, so that the legs come into play.

Stress Fracture of the Ribs. If this happens during a race the rower will not be able to stop rowing because of the rest of the crew.

First-Aid. The rower must be given a suitable support. Rib fractures can be immobilised by binding the arm to the chest with a stretch bandage. If both sides of the ribs are broken, both arms may be bound to the chest until medical help can be sought.

Abdominal Strains can result if muscles are not toned up at the start of a season. Lying back at the end of the stroke may contribute.

Rower's Cramp (tenosynovitis) is of the same origin as writer's cramp, tennis elbow and a number of similar sports injuries.

First-Aid is not very effective as once the cramp has started it is often intractable and continued rowing is bound to aggravate it. Prevention is often the only cure. If the oar is held lightly in the fingers and not gripped at any part of the stroke, especially at the finish where the twisting movement may cause trouble, it need never start – but once started, it is likely to recur unless techniques are improved. Hand and forearm exercises are the best preventive.

Injury Specific to Canoeing

Shoulder Strain. If a single paddle is used, the upper shoulder may become strained with over-use. With a double paddle both shoulders are likely to be affected. The bursa under the deltoid muscle can become inflamed.

First-Aid. Ice packs on landing, or cold compresses if ice is not available.

86

Rest is essential with at least one arm in a sling alternating if both are affected.

Injuries Specific to Yachting

Wrists or arms can be broken if the winch handle, used to turn the winch, backs up. Broken legs have also been known to occur.

First-Aid. In the case of a broken wrist or arm, the damaged limb must be immobilised immediately with a splint and sling. A makeshift splint can be made from a rolled newspaper, a flat piece of board or equivalent, and a makeshift sling from a scarf. When a leg has been broken, make the injured person comfortable and immobilise him in his bunk with straps and sandbags if the weather is rough.

Injuries Specific to Angling

In dry-fly casting a fisherman has sometimes been hooked by a fellow sportsman.

First-Aid. If the hook is embedded in the skin it must not be pulled out as the barb will tear the flesh, but pushed further through to the nearest surface. The wound must be treated as any open wound with disinfectant, sterile gauze and possibly toxoid or anti-tetanus injections. Ice, if available, or a PR spray may be used partially to anaesthetise the wound before removing the hook.

Bursitis. A wear-and-tear effect on the shoulder from frequent casting and possibly also cold and damp may cause bursitis, an inflammation of the shoulder. The bursa is a small sac between the joints filled with fluid which may become inflamed by excessive use. There is also the possibility that a hidden focus of infection or gout may aggravate the condition.

First-Aid. The pain can be acute and can only be relieved by painkillers until medical aid can be reached.

Finger Injuries. When a fish is hooked and is being played there is a danger of getting the line round a finger or ankle and this can be pulled so tight that it may cause serious injury, especially to a finger. In sea fishing, fingers are also at risk. A fisherman who puts his hand in the bucket containing the catch, perhaps to get a piece of mackerel for bait, may, if he has previously caught a conger, have his finger bitten off.

First-Aid. The severed finger or fingers should be kept on ice, the wound lightly covered with sterile gauze, a painkiller given to the patient who should be rushed off to hospital as soon as possible where it may be possible for a team of surgeons to sew the finger(s) on again.

Winter Sports: Skiing, Bob-Sledding, Ice Hockey

SKIING

Avalanches

Ski resorts are located in areas considered to be well protected from avalanches but higher slopes are vulnerable at all seasons and lower slopes particularly in spring. This being so, it is unlikely that there is danger to those taking part in any winter sport other than skiing.

Warning of avalanche conditions are usually given but every year skiers do get caught and sometimes killed by one which came suddenly or by ignoring warnings such as ski slopes marked 'closed' (or '*fermé*' or '*gesperrt*'). Falling on a suspect slope may set off the avalanche; untracked slopes should be avoided in avalanche conditions and, if they must be crossed, it is advisable to stick close to trees which can impede the snowfall.

Obviously, if caught, the skier should try to get out of the path by skiing to the side. If this fails, it is best, if possible, in a wet-snow avalanche, to get rid of the skis and keep on the surface by 'swimming'. In dry snow, cover the nose and try to push the ski stick through the surface of the snow to attract rescuers.

Rescue teams form part of all ski resorts' resources. At well organised points are sledges provided with blankets, splints and other first-aid materials waiting for an SOS telephone call which will usually be made by an experienced skier who happens to be in the neighbourhood of the accident. This skier may be the one to collect the sledge and bring it to the injured person and propel him to the village first-aid post or to the doctor's or surgeon's office. Every skier should find out just what the arrangements are for rescue near the piste as he may find himself either in the role of the experienced skier or the victim.

Other Hazards and Injuries Specific to Skiing

For British skiers the briefness of their winter holiday and the plethora of ski-lifts that have sprung up since the last war cause many difficulties.

Both result in a condition of unpreparedness. In the first case, skiers may arrive on the winter sports scene after months of non-exercising behind a desk. In the second, instead of paying for their downhill run by climbing for it – and thereby warming up all their muscles – skiers are carried up on lifts to formerly unattainable heights and ejected on to runs most probably beyond their capabilities. Instead of an hour or two's downhill skiing in a day, the inexperienced skiers, trying to make the most of their short holiday, tire their unaccustomed muscles beyond their power to serve their purpose. Serious falls at too-high speeds result and damage, mostly to legs, knees and ankles are the result of over-fatigue.

INDIRECT INJURIES

If skis get crossed, deviate or stick in soft snow, and the skier's body continues on its downward path, the lower limbs are subjected to violent twisting strains. A ligament in the knee can be badly sprained or even ruptured. Ankles can be severely sprained or the bones in the lower leg (tibia and fibula) or the ankle may fracture.

Eighty per cent of leg damage is caused by rotation strains, sprains and breaks, according to a Ski Club of Great Britain report.

A forward fall, where the ski sticks and the skier pitches forward, frequently causes tears at the back of the ankle and rupture of the tendo-Achilles and accounts for five per cent of these.

First-Aid. Differential diagnosis is impossible without diagnostic tools such as X-ray. Unless the bone is actually sticking through the flesh, it is hard to tell a strain from a sprain or a fracture. If the ankle is damaged, leave the boot on but cut the laces. Splint or immobilise the damaged area and elevate during transportation to a medical centre. The same applies to indirect injuries.

DIRECT INJURIES

Other injuries are due to the impact of one ski on the shin of the other leg. A few are caused by the direct clash with hard objects.

BOB-SLEDDING

There are no injuries specific to bob-sledding since these can include the whole range from minor contusions and bruises, ice burns, blisters at different layers, to almost any broken bone or combination of bones, to fatal injury and death. The speeds on icy runs make injury inevitable in the event of a spill or an over-run. The dangers possible when a bob-sled runs over the top of the track include striking rocks, trees or even buildings and can be very serious or quite minor according to the luck of the game. If the bob-sled overturns within the run the sledders may be dragged, possibly causing burns or other abrasions, or ejected at speed. There may then be the danger of head injuries. The possibility of a fatality is minimised by crash helmets though concussion can still happen. Multiple fractures in which the bones in an arm or leg can be broken into fragments have occasionally taken place.

First-Aid is rarely necessary as at any well-organised run on a recognised track local surgeons, expert at mending broken bones, are immediately available. One Swiss surgeon showed the authors an X-ray in which an arm was shattered into twenty-seven bone segments which he was stringing together as if it were a jigsaw puzzle. With properly applied traction and counter traction the arm recovered.

ICE HOCKEY

Damage to Teeth

Where you have well padded gladiators attacking each other with hockey sticks or using the puck as a deadly projectile, you will find many hockey players devoid of front teeth.

First-Aid. If they can be found (and they are often knocked into the victim's mouth who spits them out with blood), the broken teeth should be kept as the dentist may use them to cap the roots. American players now use a plastic mask to avoid facial damage.

Bumps, Bruises and Cuts

These may result from one player's skates being caught in the opponent's, causing both to trip on hard ice.

First-Aid. With minor degrees of contusions the player may be able to continue to play after some protection has been applied to the injured part. If the ankle or knee are painful on taking weight, the player should come off the ice as he may have a severe strain or sprain in addition to bruising. Ice, support and elevation will help until medical aid is available. Don't give a painkiller as it may obscure symptoms.

Painful Feet

Caused by the hardness of the skates and the coldness of the ice, these may cause agony across the base of the toes (the metatarsal arch) and up the sciatic nerve in the leg.

First-Aid. The boot or boots should be removed and a painkiller in this case is advisable as it may relieve the spasm. If this happens often an arch support will help, plus skating boots large enough to accomodate two pairs of thick socks. The support may consist of a sponge rubber pad. If the pain is in the tendo-Achilles at the back of the ankle, sponge-rubber padding held by strapping should be introduced into the back of the boot.

Stress Fractures

These may result in the bones at the base of the toes from the sustained force applied to the foot.

First-Aid. If the player suspects a break, the boot should be left on with the laces untied, and he should be carried by stretcher, with the leg elevated, to a medical centre.

4
The Active Therapeutic Approach to Recovery

This chapter is mainly for the medical profession but sportsmen may like to learn the whys and wherefores of their treatment and how they can help themselves to quicker recovery.

General Considerations

In sports injuries a quick recovery is often the hallmark of good treatment. Recovery time, however, depends on the correct diagnosis and the right type of treatment. Combinations of various treatments go to make up the 'Active Therapeutic Approach'. The AT Approach includes periods of rest as well as periods of activity. Instructions are given to the patient as to the exact amount of rest he must have at first, but this is combined with short, often frequent periods of exercises of a non-straining nature. An exact knowledge of these facts is of particular importance to the general practitioner and physiotherapist interested in sports injury.

There are still many who consider that apart from the application of ice and ultrasound, recovery from injury depends almost entirely on the time factor. This rather pessimistic outlook is certainly not necessarily true of the modern sportsman, who often recovers in record time, enabling him to return to his sport quite quickly.

Recovery time for activity in ordinary everyday life is often also much reduced, but the recovery times given on page 118 are those for returning to full sporting activities. There is a certain element of risk when returning to sport early which the professional sportsman is often willing to take for the sake of his career.

The orthopaedic surgeon, who has had the experience of treating many thousands of athletic injuries personally, is in the best position to give an opinion on the value of the different kinds of treatment advised. Often it will be found that many forms of physical treatment help a little each time they are applied, and it is the sum total of these improvements that eventually produces a quick recovery.

Factors Relating to the Anatomy and Pathology of Athletic Injuries

Before considering the diagnosis and treatment of each individual injury which an athlete may sustain, it is important that certain aspects in the field of anatomy, pathology and other related factors are clearly understood.

Hilton's axiom that all injuries should be treated by rest did not differentiate between those conditions in which sepsis played a major part and those in which there was no breakage of the skin or bloodstream infection. Obviously those injuries in which acute, sub-acute or chronic infections are present require absolute rest, whereas those due to injury alone will benefit by modified rest of the muscles combined with forms of exercise without strain. Provided the amount of exercise is carefully graded, it helps to keep the muscles in good condition and at the same time aids the dispersal of traumatic effusion. It also stimulates good healing of bone and soft tissue structures by the improved flow of arterial blood. Otherwise, there is stagnation of venous blood, and metabolites (waste products) are left stranded in the tissue fluids and cells. The right balance between rest and activity is essential and the right amount of each must be advised in individual cases.

Important points to be stressed and which must be thoroughly understood include:

1. Those factors responsible for the injury.
   (a) Sudden direct injury: the degree of contusion and bruising of the tissues will obviously depend on the severity of the injury from slight to severe. Even necrosis or death of the tissues may occur.
   (b) Indirect injury: strains cause stretching and even tearing of muscles and tendons, which form the first line of protection of the joints. In sprains, the capsular structures of the joint or underlying bones may be involved. Often in the case of joint injury one side is involved by the indirect injury to soft tissues, whereas the ligaments and other soft tissues on the opposite side suffer direct injury from the effects

93

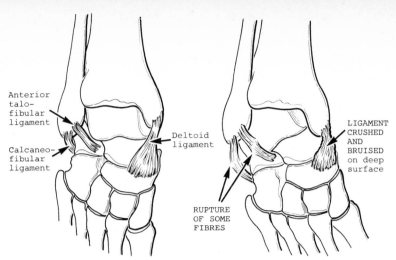

Anterior talo-fibular ligament

Calcaneo-fibular ligament

Deltoid ligament

LIGAMENT CRUSHED AND BRUISED on deep surface

RUPTURE OF SOME FIBRES

Figure 13. Indirect and direct injury to ankle. *Left* Front view of medial and lateral ligaments of right ankle. *Right* Indirect injury causes damage to lateral ligaments. Direct injury causes bruising of deep surface of medial and spring ligaments.

of crushing and bruising on them by the direct force of the bones involved.

(c) Poor posture and the wrong execution of movements have already been stressed as one of the predisposing causes of injury. Poor posture has a pathology of its own, which shows itself as a gradual accumulation of waste products in the soft tissues as so-called 'fibrositis'. This accounts for injuries occurring from fatigue or overuse when the tissues become overloaded with waste products. It would seem that the constant pumping action of the muscles, as in 'Active Alerted Posture', keeps the circulation of waste products in the extracellular and intracellular fluids in constant flow, essential materials are delivered to the various structures and at the same time metabolites (waste products) are eliminated. These are biochemical substances and cannot be seen under the microscope. On the other hand, poor inactive posture allows the stagnation of waste products in what has been called 'the fourth circulation' – that of extracellular (interstitial) and intracellular fluid circulations. The sequence of changes in the muscular and joint structures are often the result of poor posture, incorrect mechanical use of muscles and overstrain (excessive use) producing, firstly, so-called 'fibrositis' in the muscles (bio-chemical changes). Secondly, joint sprain may be caused because the strained muscles supporting that particular joint are not working properly. Here the capsular structures, ligaments,

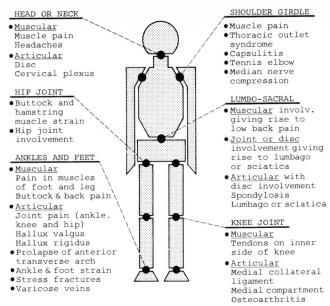

HEAD OR NECK
- Muscular
  Muscle pain
  Headaches
- Articular
  Disc
  Cervical plexus

HIP JOINT
- Buttock and
  hamstring
  muscle strain
- Hip joint
  involvement

ANKLES AND FEET
- Muscular
  Pain in muscles
  of foot and leg
  Buttock & back pain
- Articular
  Joint pain (ankle,
  knee and hip)
  Hallux valgus
  Hallux rigidus
- Prolapse of anterior
  transverse arch
- Ankle & foot strain
- Stress fractures
- Varicose veins

SHOULDER GIRDLE
- Muscle pain
- Thoracic outlet
  syndrome
- Capsulitis
- Tennis elbow
- Median nerve
  compression

LUMBO-SACRAL
- Muscular involv.
  giving rise to
  low back pain
- Joint or disc
  involvement giving
  rise to lumbago
  or sciatica
- Articular with
  disc involvement
  Spondylosis
  Lumbago or sciatica

KNEE JOINT
- Muscular
  Tendons on inner
  side of knee
- Articular
  Medial collateral
  ligament
  Medial compartment
  Osteoarthritis

Figure 14. The effects of postural strain at the six fixing levels. Progressive strain shows firstly as so called fibrositis or muscular rheumatism proceeding as age advances to joint degeneration and the onset of osteoarthritis.

synovial membrane, and finally the joint epichondrium (end of bone), become involved. Thirdly, as soon as fibrillation of this takes place, osteoarthritis (osteoarthrosis) begins.

(d) If a muscle contracts and an opposing force suddenly checks the movement, there is a danger that the muscle will tear or rupture.

(e) Very occasionally in athletes there may be an unsuspected pathological factor present which converts a trivial injury into a serious one – that is, a cyst in the bone causing a pathological fracture.

2. Important factors in the anatomy and pathology of injuries related to treatment.

(a) The spread of traumatic effusion is not only influenced by the arrangement of the tissue planes and the forces of gravity, but also by muscle action and the direction of the flow of blood and lymph.

(b) The extensibility and contractibility (flexibility) of the muscular structures must be maintained by graduated exercises. These allow for full extension and flexion in joint movement.

(c) At all costs the blood supply to the injured structures must not be impeded. If there is any danger of death of the tissues from exces-

95

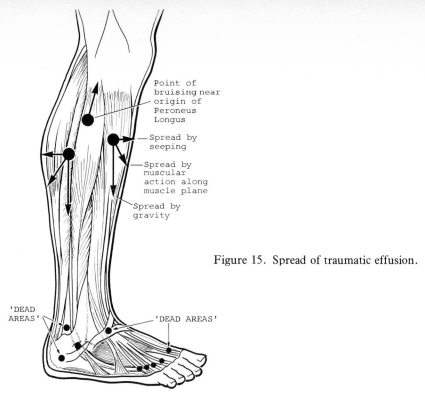

Point of
bruising near
origin of
Peroneus
Longus

Spread by
seeping

Spread by
muscular
action along
muscle plane

Spread by
gravity

'DEAD
AREAS'

'DEAD AREAS'

Figure 15. Spread of traumatic effusion.

sive pressure either on the arterial or venous side, immediate relief
of this pressure must be a paramount necessity by operation or by
the removal of any compressing force, such as a tight bandage or
plaster cast.

(d) Often the recovery from injuries near joints is slow because of the
involvement of neighbouring bursae. This may be due to pressure
or rubbing on the bursa from friction of an overlying muscle or by a
bony structure inside. Both may cause a type of recurring attrition
injury to an overlying tendon. If the athlete has a gouty tendency the
bursae around the joint may be affected and this may be a further
factor in maintaining symptoms.

(e) Articular cartilage varies in individuals and in different joints. It
consists mainly of chondrotin sulphuric acid and collagen fibres. In
weight-bearing bones chondrotin sulphuric acid predominates
where strength is needed, whereas for resilience in the upper
extremity joints there is a greater proportion of collagen fibres.

(f) Injury affects the normal manufacture of synovial fluid which is a
viscid and slippery substance derived by dialysis of plasma from the

96

blood and tissue fluids. Excessive stimulation by injury or too much exercise may produce a synovial effusion (synovitis).

3. Traumatic syndromes, phases and stages.

The negative and positive phases of wound healing and recovery are well known. At first, according to the severity of the injury, if there is a varying amount of damaged tissue with blood effusion and traumatic oedema, the positive healing phase will not take place until the damaged or dead tissues and traumatic swelling are removed or absorbed. The negative phases last until this occurs, but can be accelerated, in many cases by the evacuation of these by aspiration, or adequate incision and expression. By the stroke of a knife the negative phase can be transformed into the positive healing phase. These phases correspond with the acute, sub-acute and chronic stages in the course of recovery from an injury. The latter chronic stage should never occur if the Active Therapeutic Approach to injury is applied.

Figure 16. Positive and negative phases of healing in capsulitis of the shoulder.

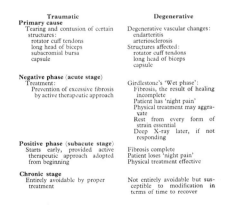

Traumatic	Degenerative
Primary cause	
Tearing and contusion of certain structures:	Degenerative vascular changes:
rotator cuff tendons	endarteritis
long head of biceps	arteriosclerosis
subacromial bursa	Structures affected:
capsule	rotator cuff tendons
	long head of biceps
	capsule
Negative phase (acute stage)	
Treatment:	Girdlestone's 'Wet phase':
Prevention of excessive fibrosis by active therapeutic approach	Fibrosis, the result of healing incomplete
	Patient has 'night pain'
	Physical treatment may aggravate
	Rest from every form of strain essential
	Deep X-ray later, if not responding
Positive phase (subacute stage)	
Starts early, provided active therapeutic approach adopted from beginning	Fibrosis complete
	Patient loses 'night pain'
	Physical treatment effective
Chronic stage	
Entirely avoidable by proper treatment	Not entirely avoidable but susceptible to modification in terms of time to recover

4. There are certain factors pertaining to either the cause or the effect of injury.

(a) Environment: changes in temperatures—excessive heat or cold and draughts – are often detrimental to injured structures or may in themselves precipitate a pathological state.

(b) Circulation: estimation of the circulation of the injured part should always be made, and the question asked: have the arterial, venous or lymphatic circulations been involved in any way by injury?

(c) Infection and toxic conditions: obviously the presence of infection will influence healing, and in the older athlete, if an injury is not getting better quickly, there is always the possibility of gout.

(d) Accident proneness: many people are accident prone, but by attention to Active Alerted Posture they may be able to overcome this tendency by becoming aware of the correct way to distribute weight on their joints and by learning how they should always make their actions work on a firm base.

(e) Psychosomatic: it is only occasionally that athletes will show functional disability. It may be that they realise they are not up to the high standards of certain athletic achievements and therefore make their injury an excuse for not getting better or being unable to compete. However, if this is realised by the doctor and trainer it may be possible to give advice about certain special training exercises which will help to strengthen their particular weakness. Thus a different approach to training may be important.

(f) Friction or attrition of a bony, cartilaginous or fibrous thickening may cause pressure and gradually fray or even cause a structure such as a tendon to rupture: that is, the long head of biceps tendon (at the front of the shoulder). Constant pressure, as from fibrous bands, may be the cause of the various entrapment syndromes affecting nerves throughout the body. It would seem that fibrous bands can form in many places in the body and cause pressure.

(g) Other factors (Helal, 1975) influencing accidents are: fatigue; inexperience; poor technique; uncontrolled speed; poor snow (in the case of snow skiing); poor visibility; and in water skiing, lack of proper care on the part of the driver of the ski-boat and lack of awareness by other drivers and skiers in the vicinity.

5. There are certain fundamental factors associated with athletic injuries which have an effect on recovery.

(a) The amount of traumatic swelling. If a blood vessel is broken, the amount of haematoma (a collection of blood forming a swelling) may be enormous, especially in certain parts of the body where the tissues are loose and slack, such as the scrotal region and around the eyes.

(b) The components of traumatic swelling. All four circulations may be involved: arterial, venous, lymphatic and tissue fluid, and if the synovial membrane of a joint, tendon or bursa is stimulated, there may be synovial effusion as well. It is when it is in the fluid state that absorption is easier and quicker, so that the immediate AT Approach has a chance of producing a quick recovery. This is accomplished either by aspiration, evacuation or by stimulating absorption through intensive physiotherapy including exercises and manipulations. The exercises may, of course, in the early stages have to be non-weight-bearing or non-strain ones with intervals of limb elevation and complete rest in between.

(c) The phenomenon of the spread or seeping of traumatic effusion is a most interesting one and it is governed by the force of gravity, the direction of tissue planes, blood vessels and muscular action. Owing to the convergence of tissue planes in certain parts of the body, a collection of the components of traumatic effusion may tend to form thickenings and adhesions unless quickly dispersed by the AT Approach. Also, tender thickenings may form in what have been called 'dead areas', where there is no muscular movement, as around both sides of the os calcis (the heel bone). See Figure 15, page 96.

(d) Unless dispersed quickly, large haematoma in various parts of the body may cause complications. Often these have been observed in athletes months or even years later.

(e) Muscle wasting: this can occur in the course of a few days and must be prevented at all costs by graduated exercises; if the limb is in a plaster cast, isometric exercises against the resistance of the rigid cast should be carried out for periods of five minutes every two hours if possible.

(f) Nerve involvement: it is obvious that if an injury damages a nerve, especially a motor one, the recovery time will depend largely on the severity of the involvement.

(g) Effects of the injury on the joints above and below the site of injury. Many muscles work and influence the movements of more than one joint. For example, in an injury to the knee, muscles and tendons may be damaged so that if allowed to become stiffened and shortened will not only affect the movements of the knee but also of the hip and ankle, according to whether the muscles above or below the knee are involved. This rule applies to the elbow and many other joints.

(h) Composition of fibrous thickenings. Normal fibrous tissue is made up of long molecules composed of fully extended chains of carbon and nitrogen atoms. The chains are connected by lateral linkages of carbon and nitrogen bonds. When frequent injury occurs, fibrous tissue nodules composed of disorientated fibres become mixed up in a homogenous mass. The chief aim of all treatment, including physiotherapy and injections, is to produce local oedema so that the tight mass of fibrous thickening can be softened and remoulded.

(i) Tissue tenderness. The products of tissue injury contain substances which can make the tissues tender; in the case where a haemorrhage has occurred, a substance called haemosiderin in the blood is thought to be the causative substance. It is also interesting to note that as the products of injury disperse and seep through the tissues far remote from the initial injury these may become tender and discoloured, for example, down the calf and around the ankle in quadriceps and hamstring injuries.

The combined phenomena of tissue tenderness and seepage is illustrated in the appearance of synovitis of the knee (fluid under the knee cap) occurring some days after contusion bruising of the quadriceps in the mid-thigh. Each day tenderness will appear nearer the knee joint until suddenly the knee begins to swell with synovial effusion and the surrounding tissues become tender. This synovial effusion can be explained by the irritation of the synovial membrane on its outer surface from the seeping of the products of bruising down the thigh to the upper part of the knee joint. Another explanation is that the serum in the haematoma seeps down the thigh and through the synovial membrane into the joint causing synovial swelling. Possibly it is a combination of both.

(j) If one group of muscles is strained, tenderness often occurs in the opposite antagonistic group. For example, if the groin adductors (inside of thigh) are strained or torn it is important to treat the corresponding antagonistic abductors, the glutei (buttock muscles). It would seem that the normal metabolism of the antagonistic muscles is disturbed with the production of waste products in them and these cause tissue tenderness. This is probably due to loss of muscle balance between the two groups.

100

Examination, Diagnosis and Preliminary Treatment

After the best possible first-aid, the injured athlete may have to be transported to the nearest treatment centre. The surgeon in charge will, if necessary, have him admitted.

A thorough examination of the patient must be carried out immediately so as to give an accurate diagnosis. Sometimes the surgeon may only be able to make a general one, such as a certain type of fracture, a sprained joint, a contusion, bruise or tearing of muscles. Before a complete diagnosis is possible he must take an exact history of the accident, how and when it occurred and other factors relevant to it, such as the time and type of day it was, dry or rainy. Each part of the sportsman's actions up to the injury should be studied and analysed by the surgeon to ascertain whether they were carried out correctly. A study of this analysis is often rewarding as it reminds the surgeon at a later date during rehabilitation to correct the athlete's actions if they have been wrongly executed, thus enabling him to avoid recurrence in the future.

The patient may be brought in unconscious and the story of what happened to cause his injury must be extracted in as much detail as possible from the first-aid assistants. This detailed history should also include previous injuries, diseases, family history and occupation in everyday life.

An accurate examination includes observation of the site of injury: the skin temperature of the injured region, tender points or areas, swellings, soft, hard or bony. The range of movements, active, passive, assisted and against resistance, are carefully noted and compared with those of the opposite side. The surgeon often decides on further investigations and the following should be included:

1. *X-rays.* Films in several planes may be required. Anterior, posterior, lateral, obliques and, in the case of the knee, tunnel and axial views. If strained or torn ligaments are suspected, some of the films may be taken with stress thrown on the injured ligaments to ascertain whether there is opening of the joint on the side of the injured ligament. If this is so, joint instability is almost certain to follow if not adequately treated.

2. *Special views obtained by arthrography.* These are taken after a quantity of opaque liquid, with or without air, is injected into the joint. After he

has seen the results of all these investigations, the surgeon can probably make a more exact diagnosis. If the injury is not of a simple nature he may later decide on the following further investigations in order to be able to make a more specific diagnosis.

3. *Arthroscopy*. This method of investigation is becoming increasingly popular and important. Even the small joints can be inspected with a filament lens after inserting an arthroscope into the joint under local or preferably general anaesthetic.

4. *Complete blood analysis.*

5. *Localisation of tender points* by faradic stimulation of the muscles.

After diagnosis, detailed instructions are given by the surgeon to the nursing staff and the patient as to the right amount and degree of rest and movement.

The injured part usually requires protection and support by suitable bandaging and splintage. If good support is necessary, it should be in the form of a plaster of Paris cast. A removable cast split down the front which can then be taken off for home treatment and physiotherapy is often employed. Aspiration or expression of excess traumatic effusion by incision may be necessary in the case of marked swelling of the soft tissues and joints.

6. *Pathological findings* of a section of synovial membrane or changes in synovial fluid.

ICE. These initials stand for Ice, Compression and Elevation, and these three forms of treatment are considered by many to be all that is necessary for the first forty-eight hours. Firm compression and elevation should be as continuous as possible. The treatment is necessary to prevent further exudation of fluid into the tissues and to help diminish the swelling and reaction to injury, and is as follows. *Ice* packs should be applied periodically for twenty minutes, four to six times each day. *Compression*: the well known method (Robert Jones) of wrapping the injured part in layers of wool or gamgee, with firm bandages, is the best, as the amount of compression can be easily regularised. *Elevation* can be accomplished by raising the end of the bed on blocks; by hanging the arm up (if this is involved) on a blood transfusion stand; or by placing the leg on pillows or cushions.

However, other forms of treatment may be considered necessary in addition to these three during the first forty-eight hours. These include a combination of two of the following at each treatment: wax baths, faradism, short-wave, ultrasound, micro-wave or interferential, two or three times a day according to the urgency for recovery. Between treatments isometric exercises are essential for five minutes each hour while ICE is carried out.

Heinz Kowalski, who in his younger days was a famous circus acrobat, does not think physicians treated contusions, sprains and strains very well because they always wrapped them in bandages, or immobilised them in plaster for three weeks, whereas necessity taught him that hot water soaks, rubbing with alcohol and carrying out gentle active movements made them better in twelve hours, so that he was able to continue his performances the next day. Henry Cooper, the famous boxer, substantiates this.

As the products of injury seep and spread through the tissues there may be increased swelling. It is this that makes some people cautious of AT Approach in the first forty-eight hours. However, with care and understanding, cases which seem hopeless at first can benefit out of all recognition by the immediate application of this approach. The initial swelling of the tissues near the site of the injury is essential for quick recovery as it is part of the process of seeping and subsequent easy absorption of the traumatic effusion as it becomes more superficial, especially when it surfaces into the subcutaneous pannicular tissue. Occasionally the swelling may become so tense that a session of physiotherapy may have to be missed, but ICE, with exercises during the elevation, must be continued. In addition the tension in the tissue may become so great in some cases that operative relief of this tension is necessary.

Some of the treatments commenced in first-aid must be continued or supplemented.

Surgical Treatment. Surgical intervention in athletic injuries should be advised only when the conditions for operation are superb. Sometimes the tissues are so badly contused with septic abrasions and marked general swelling that it may be advisable to wait for a few days before operating and before transporting the patient to a safe centre.

Types of cases requiring operation are:

1. Where swelling of the tissues is due to a localised haematoma, or to a general contusion and swelling of the soft tissues causing pressure on either the venous or arterial side of the circulation. Circulatory disturbance of this nature occurs in the tissues around the elbow and forearm and in the front of the lower leg and unless relieved by decompression can

very quickly lead to the death of the muscles. Examples – Volkmann's ischaemia of the elbow and forearm muscles and necrosis of the muscles of the anterior tibial compartment in front of the leg below the knee.

2. Contusions and fractures of the skull to arrest intracranial pressure and even save life.

3. Compound wounds and compound fractures with open soft tissue wounds leading to the fracture site require immediate removal of all ragged, badly contused and dead tissues, including, in the case of fractures, small separate pieces of bone, which have become so detached that they have lost their blood supply.

4. Certain chest and abdominal wounds, especially where there has been injury to vital intrathoracic (chest) and abdominal structures.

5. Unstable fractures and dislocations requiring stabilisation in a plaster of Paris cast or by means of intramedullary nails, plates and screws, pins or wires.

6. Tears of intra-articular structures such as the meniscii of the knee with or without damage of ligaments.

Delayed operations. Where there is extensive bruising and contusion of the soft tissue with evidence of sepsis near the major site of injury, it is advisable to postpone operation for several days. Much of the traumatic swelling can be absorbed by elevation, non weight-bearing exercises, contrast baths and physiotherapy. A definitive operation, such as plating of a fracture or intramedullary nailing, must not be carried out near the presence of sepsis.

This also applies when the tissues are badly contused and bruised. Occasionally, however, particularly in injuries to the hand and foot, contusion bruising may be so severe that it may be wise to make a series of small incisions into the tissues to allow expression and seepage of the traumatic effusions, otherwise extensive blistering with possible skin loss may prevent or make difficult further necessary operative procedures which normally would be carried out a few days after the accident.

Here is an example. A severe fracture dislocation of the foot at the mid-tarsal joints was complicated by extensive bruising and contusion of the soft tissues. The leg and foot were placed in light plaster support without reducing the fractures and dislocation. Three days later at operation it was found that there was so much blistering of the skin that operative open reduction of the fractures and dislocations was still impossible. Early operation should always apply to cases where there is a danger of involvement of the skin from subsequent blistering resulting from seepage of traumatic effusion from deeper structures.

Sportsmen as a rule should be retained in hospital after an operation until the wound is one-hundred-per-cent healed. If they are allowed to leave hospital before the stitches are removed, and good wound healing has been accomplished, there is often the likelihood of their doing something stupid such as exercising too vigorously. This allows the wound area to become excessively swollen with possible breaking open of the wound. It will pay every time to be adamant that they should not be out of good supervision until the wound is soundly healed. *This cannot be stressed too strongly.* If anything tends to go wrong with wound healing it is often because the sportsman is too anxious to get back in record time. However, the surgeon must not be complacent and every form of treatment employed under the AT Approach must be employed so that the sportsman is confident that everything is being carried out to hasten his full recovery. This is where instructions about regular periods of exercises during the day with the help of a good physiotherapist make all the difference.

Treatment by the Physiotherapist

The surgeon must give exact instructions to the physiotherapist as to the type of treatment required, such as the various methods of massage and the strength that should be employed, the use of wax baths, ultrasound, short-wave, faradism, interferential current, micro-wave and manipulative treatment.

Very gentle manipulative movements are performed daily without an anaesthetic during the early stages and later it may be necessary to carry them out more strenuously under a general anaesthetic if movements are not progressing and are still painful if forced. Often the physiotherapist will note changes in physical signs and symptoms from day to day and the surgeon should be informed about these observations as it may be necessary to make slight alterations in the treatment programme.

In the same way as many types of drugs have different effects on individuals requiring medical treatment, the reactions to different forms of physical treatment vary in individuals. During a routine case, the types of physical treatment are often varied, as many as three or four types being given during one treatment lasting three-quarters of an hour. If necessary, the patient is given two sessions each day, and of course he should carry out his home treatment several times daily.

Home treatment by the patient should be taught him by the specialist and re-checked by the physiotherapist, who will make sure that he is doing every part of it correctly.

Recovery Time. Many athletes also have no idea of the necessary time it takes for an injury to recover. This applies particularly to fractures as an athlete will often be convinced that a fracture of both tibia and fibula with displacement, requiring either an open operation or plaster immobilisation, will be consolidated sufficiently to allow full activity in six weeks, whereas to restore it fully in four months is quick and depends on the setting and healing of the bone, muscles and circulatory system being first-rate.

Help by the Trainer. The trainer is often brought in as soon as the injured athlete is able to bear weight on an injured lower limb. In certain cases the trainer and the physiotherapist may work together. In fact, in some professional clubs the injured athlete may have as many as four different types of physiotherapy during a morning's session; in between treatments the physiotherapist will pass him on to the trainer, who will give him light exercises at first but graduate quickly to a more strenuous programme if there is no undue reaction, such as pain or swelling.

Some trainers insist that the player, when injured in the leg muscles, although he may stop his sport, must keep on jogging so as to prevent the torn muscle contracting. Obviously he must not stand about getting cold, and most doctors would advise an immediate shower and rub down, followed by ice packs, compression by wool and bandage, and elevation of the injured limb.

Various Forms of Therapy

After diagnosis of any injury, the AT Approach, including home treatment, is applied so that every appropriate form of physical treatment can be administered several times daily if required. Only by adhering strictly to this regime will recovery take place in the shortest possible time. In the early stages periods of complete rest may be indicated, but these can be combined with increasingly longer periods of activity.

Before considering the various forms of treatment, it is important to keep in mind the objects to be aimed at in treatment. The injured structures must be restored to as near normal as before the accident. To accomplish this all injured muscles, tendons, and soft tissues must be returned to their former resilience, extensibility and flexibility. Muscles often waste and become atonic after injury and must be made strong, fully restored in bulk as well as strength. If fractures have occurred the accurate alignment, length and structure of the fractured bones must be restored to as near normal as possible and the joints above and below the site of injury rehabilitated to full movement and muscle power.

In treating any part of the arm each joint right up to the neck must be included. For example, if the wrist is injured there is often some degree of involvement of the elbow, shoulder and neck structures, caused by the injury, jarring the other joints. The same principle also applies to the leg. Injuries involving the knee joint can affect the muscles and soft tissue of the ankle, hip joints and lumbo-sacral spine. Treatment must therefore include all structures right up to the lumbo-sacral spine at waist level.

The extent of traumatic effusion must first be minimised by ICE (see p. 102). Movements and resilience of the muscles and other soft tissues are restored by graduated exercises and physiotherapy. All these methods go to make up the AT Approach.

Sometimes the injured structure is only returned to eighty per cent of normal which allows sufficient function for everyday life.

In moderate degrees of exercise such as are required for sports like tennis or golf of a non-competitive nature, function of the injured part must be restored to about ninety per cent. However, for the vigorous participation needed in first-class competitive sport one-hundred-per-cent fitness is essential. It is therefore imperative for a sportsman of international standard to make a full, perfect recovery before again participating in his activity. After an accurate assessment of the injury the surgeon will probably advise a course of physiotherapy. It would seem appropriate, then, at this stage to give a few details of the different forms of physiotherapy he may recommend. These are: massage; manipulation; cold therapy; heat therapy, superficial and deep; interferential therapy; faradism; injection techniques; proprioceptive neuromuscular facilitation exercises (PNF).

1. MASSAGE

It would seem there is a great deal of confusion as to the role of massage and manipulative treatment in recent injury. Many physiotherapists have the impression that the teaching and employment of massage have been given up. In the physiotherapist's curriculum, massage techniques are relegated to the pre-manipulative treatment – that is to say, in preparing the muscles and restoring them to their full extensibility – so that when the manipulative techniques are carried out they are not impeded by muscle spasm and shortening.

The whole field of massage is covered by effleurage (stroking), petrissage (kneading), tapôtment (percussion, striking, vibration and shaking), and friction (rubbing). The good physiotherapist appreciates which is the right type of massage for each case. He must consider the age and type of patient he is treating. Strong young athletes may require deep friction and kneading, whereas these might be hurtful and damaging to the older patient whose tissues are inclined to be tender. Some form of massage cream is usually employed to lessen skin resistance.

It is easy to discern the good physiotherapist because he combines rhythmic kneading massage and the exact amount of firmness and depth with short periods of deep friction. Many are inclined to rub hard, moving the skin and underlying pannicular tissues painfully on the muscle and deeper structures. In good massage, muscular spasm is overcome with the restoration of muscle length, resilience and extensibility and this preparation of the muscles must be an integral part of manipulative techniques as stressed by Alan Stoddard.

2. MANIPULATIVE AND MOBILISATION TECHNIQUES

The techniques employed in manipulations are often not carried out in sequence, as the manipulator sometimes has the impression that they consist of simply putting the joint through a full range of movements under anaesthesia. The object of all manipulative treatment in recent injury is, firstly, to maintain the resilience of all the soft tissue, in the case of the muscles, their extensibility and flexibility (contractibility); secondly, to prevent adhesion formation. This is the reason for advising gentle mobilisation techniques as part of the daily physiotherapeutic regime for recent injuries. When the soft tissues, including the muscles, have been allowed to become stiff, manipulative measures are then intro-

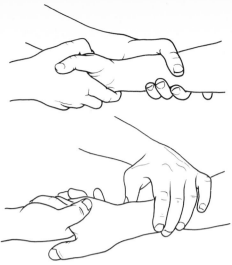

Figure 17. Manipulation Principle I. Traction and counter-traction. This stretches the capsule ligaments and other soft tissues, helping to restore their resilience.

Figure 18. Manipulation Principle II. Carrying out involuntary accessory or joint-play movements. The carpus and hand are carried to the little finger side by the right hand of the manipulator while the thumb of the left hand and other fingers are drawing and pushing the wrist to the thumb side.

duced to restore their resilience. Manipulations can take place either without an anaesthetic, with an anaesthetic, or following the mobilisation techniques taught by Maitland.

In the 1920s and 30s James Mennell did the medical profession an enormous service by postulating that all manipulative techniques must consist of three definite and separate principles.

Principle I is simply distracting the joint by holding the bones and soft tissues to be manipulated with one hand proximal to the joint to be manipulated, and pulling or distracting the distal part with the other hand, so that the joint surfaces are separated. This has the effect of restoring the resilience of the capsule and soft tissues as well as separating the bony structures. With the larger joints, an assistant may be needed to hold firm the limb above the joint to be manipulated, so as to allow the manipulator himself to use two hands for distracting the joint by traction from below. At first this distraction of the joint surface should be carried out in slight joint flexion.

Principle II. The involuntary, accessory movements are carried out as described by James Mennell. His son John calls these movements 'joint play movements'. While traction and counter-traction are applied, the accessory movements which restore the gliding rotatory side-bending movements of one bone on another are executed.

In manipulating the wrist joint, for example, the ulna and radius are held firmly above while the carpal bones and hand are moved sideways, first to the thumb side and then to the little finger side. These movements are still followed with traction and counter-traction applied, moving the

109

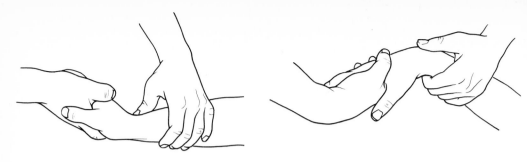

Figure 19. Manipulation Principle III.

whole carpus and hand backwards and forwards on the ulna and radius. Finally, twisting and side-bending movements of the carpus and hand on the ulna and radius are performed. The full range of involuntary accessory joint-play movements should be restored before the final manoeuvre can be performed. The restoration to normal of these joint-play movements in the second principle constitutes the movements carried out in the mobilisation techniques. A slight gradual increase of movements is obtained each day.

Principle III. In these movements the joint surfaces are separated by traction and counter-traction at the same time as the joint is put through its full range of active movements up to the point of pain. The distal bone of the joint is levered forwards in flexion whereas the proximal bone or bones are pushed backwards. The opposite takes place in extension – that is, the distal bone is levered backwards while the proximal bone is pushed forwards.

Manipulation of Muscles Which Have Been Allowed to Shorten

Firstly, the proximal end of the muscle is fixed with one hand and, secondly, the distal end is moved from side to side, at the same time stretching the muscle to restore its resiliency. Sometimes in capsulitis of

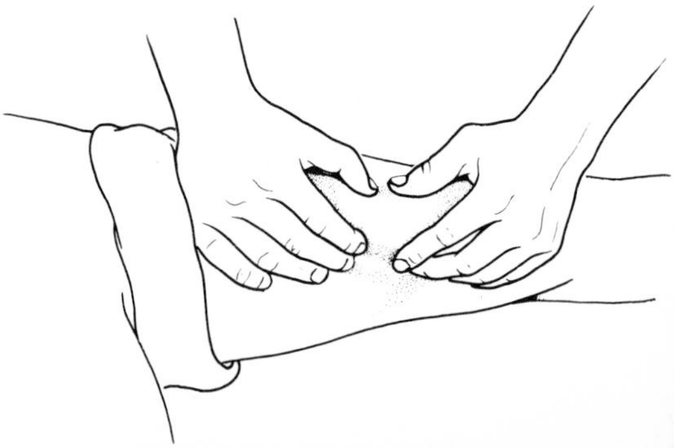

Figure 20. Manipulation for shortened muscle.

110

the shoulder it is most important first of all to restore the full length of the muscles before breaking down adhesions.

These procedures can all be carried out gently without an anaesthetic, but in some cases when complete relaxation is required they must be performed under a general anaesthetic. For instance, where there has been a history of recent injury at least a month previously and there is definite limitation of movement in one direction only, it is sometimes quicker to break adhesions and free the accessory joint-play movements by manipulation under an anaesthetic. This should be followed by further physiotherapy, including gentle manipulation again. There are also cases which, in spite of regular gentle manipulations, get to a point where movements stop short of full range and these cases usually require a manipulation under a general anaesthetic to restore the last few degrees.

In manipulative treatment there are certain rules which must be strictly adhered to, especially if it is performed under general anaesthesia. These are:

1. An exact diagnosis must be made.

2. Radiographic examination should always be carried out.

3. The phase or stage through which the condition is passing at the time must be realised. It must be in the positive healing phase before manipulation under a general anaesthetic is contemplated.

4. Any toxic or septic condition must be eliminated before manipulations are performed.

5. A reaction with pain when the patient becomes conscious, especially if the manipulation is carried out under general anaesthetic, is likely, but if local injections are given into areas where adhesions have been broken, the reaction and pain should not last longer than forty-eight hours.

6. Always see that the joints above and below the joint manipulated have their full range of movements.

7. Even if performed under general anaesthesia, no undue force must be applied. Gentle handling of the tissues must be carried out and a long lever should never be used.

The third principle in manipulative techniques should never be employed until the joint is improving. Otherwise muscle spasm is present and the manipulative movements will only aggravate the joint and produce protective spasm.

In the third technique, when the joint is ready, movements of low intensity but with high velocity should be employed and adhesions will be felt to give.

111

8. First-class ancillary physiotherapy is useful after manipulation. Several forms of physiotherapy are employed with home treatment, postural training and injections.

9. Manipulation under general anaesthesia should be left to the specialist in the field.

Maitland's mobilisation techniques are described as being of small amplitude and the speed of the movement is such that the patient cannot prevent it taking place. There are four grades of movement from a small range movement at the beginning of the range (Grade I) to a large range movement performed to the limit of the range (Grade III) and a small range movement at the end of the range (Grade IV). The type of manipulations are influenced by the different presentation of pain, muscle spasm and physical resistance.

3. COLD THERAPY

The object of this treatment is to constrict blood vessels so as to modify the amount of swelling and to lessen pain. Therefore, cold therapy is used particularly in the first forty-eight hours after the injury. Methods of carrying this out are:

Ice packs. Cubes of ice wrapped in a face-cloth or plastic bag.
Sprays. Ethyl chloride; PR (Boots); Skefron (Smith, Kline, French); cold-water sprays.

There is also a secondary superficial dilatation which is helpful before PNF exercises are given.

4. HEAT THERAPY

Superficial: infra-red radiation; molten wax; heat pads; poultices;
Deep: short-wave diathermy; micro-wave therapy; ultrasound.

Infra-red Radiation

Various forms of heat lamps: radiant heat; infra-red heat.

Some doctors are against heat in the case of brachial neuritis and sciatica. However, if it is combined with cold compresses or ice packs, and ultrasound, pain will be relieved to a greater extent.

Molten Wax

Wax baths, with thermostatic control to keep the wax at a constant temperature, help to soften inflammatory thickenings.

Heat Pads

Hot wet towels, wrung out before application. Electrical heat pads. Hot water bottles. They all have a sedative effect helping to reduce pain.

Poultices

Antiphlogistine, Kaolin. Method of application: warm the tin for two minutes in hot water; spread some of the contents on to a piece of lint as if you were buttering bread; cover with a piece of gauze to prevent it sticking to the skin; heat before a fire or on a saucer over a pan of boiling water; test against the back of the hand before applying; cover with cottonwool, oilskin and bandage. A ready-prepared poultice (Medilintex) may be used instead.

Short-wave Diathermy

This is a form of heat therapy which induces within the tissues a current of such high frequency that no electrical sensation is experienced by the patient. It induces vaso-dilation and increases blood flow, thus helping to absorb the products of traumatic swellings. In recent injuries and neuritis it is important to employ a sub-thermal dose.

In recent injuries short-wave is tending to be employed less than previously as compared to ultrasound as the strength of its application is difficult to gauge.

Micro-wave Therapy

Similar in its effect to short-wave and it has only one electrode, but the depth of penetration is less.

Ultrasound Therapy

Ultrasound waves are produced from the treatment head of the ultrasound machine by vibration of a crystal of quartz or similar material. These sound waves, which have a much higher frequency than the sound waves we can hear, have three effects: they produce heat in the tissues through which they pass; they increase the rate of flow of fluids between the tissues; they have an analgesic effect (lessening pain). The sound waves heat the ligaments, tendons and joints more than the muscles. Therefore this method is useful in the treatment of joint sprains and strains. Those waves employed are in accoustic frequency of about 27.700,000, and by producing chemical and thermal effects in the tissue, help to reduce traumatic oedema. Ultrasound is now one of the safest and most efficient methods employed for the treatment of recent injuries as the amount of heat generated can be accurately gauged.

5. INTERFERENTIAL THERAPY

Low-frequency currents are produced in the tissues without stimulation of the skin. Two medium-frequency currents of constant intensity are applied separately and simultaneously to the skin at right angles to each other. The intensity of the combined current increases and decreases rhythmically. Where the currents meet within the body a medium-frequency current is produced, which changes its intensity in a low-frequency beat rhythm. These low-frequency intensity changes have a stimulating action inside the body. They produce an analgesic effect and allow non-weight-bearing exercises to be carried out with less pain.

6. FARADISM

This is a low-frequency current which produces small shocks usually at intervals of one to two seconds. The faradic current (named for its discoverer, Faraday, over a hundred years ago) was popularised as a form of treatment before the First World War by the late Morton Smart and Rowley Bristowe and was perfected between the wars. They would be horrified if they could see the methods of faradism these days. Faradic treatment can be harmful if the two electrodes are strapped on in fixed position and the muscles stimulated by a metronome. The same muscle fibres contract each time and tire quickly and the treatment can do more harm than good.

Smart and Bristowe taught that the only effective way to carry out faradic contradictions is to 'surge' with one hand and apply the active electrode with the other (the 'labile' method). In this way the muscles do not tire and their tone improves.

Every injured muscle has its own rate of contracting and relaxing. If the

114

physiotherapist passes from one muscle to another, giving each five to six contractions, there is no chance he will tire any one muscle, and if a core stimulator is employed each muscle can be made to contract to just the amount that is comfortable and beneficial. The mechanical way of regulating the rate of stimulation to each muscle does not take into consideration the special condition of each individual muscle as regards its stage in recovery.

Faradism is scarcely used in general physiotherapy today though it is extensively used in treating horses, and in beauty parlours for slimming (spot reduction). It is still considered important in the early stages after injury where the muscles need exercise but the active contraction of muscles is too painful for the patient.

Many doctors consider that active exercises are better than the time spent on faradic stimulation of muscles. However, active exercise stimulates group movement of muscles whereas the correct method of stimulating muscles by faradism stimulates each muscle individually, thus separating one muscle from another, because in injury they often become adherent to each other.

7. INJECTION THERAPY

Injections are given for various reasons. Firstly, to produce an anaesthetic effect by blocking painful impulses or reflex disturbances such as protective muscle spasm. Secondly, to help break down granulation (inflammatory) tissue and adhesions. Thirdly, to introduce an anti-inflammatory fluid such as hydrocortisone, which has an anti-flammatory action and at the same time also increases the permeability of the blood vessels to allow quicker absorption. Fourthly, to produce a state of hyperaemia. Fifthly, to spread the reactions of manipulative techniques, free surfaces which are adherent, and promote quick absorption.

It is important to appreciate the various types of tissue reaction to injury. It is considered, as stated previously, that simple muscle strain from poor posture and the incorrect exertion of muscular action will allow deposition of metabolites or waste products in the tissues. If there is definite injury, strain, sprain or fracture, there will be an exudation of fluid in the damaged tissues which will soon form granulation tissue, in which the natural, normal arrangement of the collagen fibres of the muscles and connective tissues are disturbed. Instead of well-orientated fibres they

115

become a swollen plastic mass. Before local anaesthesia was employed many surgeons used sterile water to break up the abnormal areas. Later procaine or novocaine anaesthesia was added to the injection fluid.

Just before the Second World War lactic acid, combined with procaine, become popular. Since 1945 Laughton Scott solution of procaine, urea and salicylic acid has been employed extensively, especially after manipulation under anaesthesia, where the reaction may be painful for forty-eight hours. As much as 20 ml of one per cent xylocaine and 2 ml of Depomedrone may be employed to help lessen pain and promote the quick absorption of the reaction after the breaking down of adhesions. Recently, long-acting xylocaine (half to one per cent) has been employed on its own or in combination with other analgesics.

Some authorities recommend two per cent xylocaine, but occasionally general reactions to this strength have produced serious after-effects. Hydrocortisone as Depomedrone 1–2 ml of 40 mg in each millilitre is combined with one per cent xylocaine and injected into tender areas. An enzyme to promote quick absorption can be added, but unless mixed with one per cent xylocaine the reaction can be very painful.

Many surgeons are against the injection of hydrocortisone into joints, but it has been found that if no more than four injections are given at weekly intervals, and the patient carries out vigorous home treatment and has appropriate physiotherapy, osteochondral necrosis does not take place. A sportsman is rarely allergic to hydrocortisone, and of course it should not be given even locally if there is a history of an active gastric ulcer or haemorrhoids.

8. PROPRIOCEPTIVE NEUROMUSCULAR FACILITATION (PNF)

This is a technique perfected in the United States of America with the aim of stimulating responses in the neuromuscular mechanism and thereby improving them. The brain does not recognise individual muscles but only gross patterns of movement: isolated muscle contraction has to be learned or acquired. When muscles are injured they may have to relearn the pattern.

When this technique was first practised muscles were put through their range of movements using maximal resistance supplied by the therapist during repeated contractions. Later the range of movement was increased

116

to allow for two separate movements of each muscle group – for example, both flexion and extension of the foot instead of only flexion. The stretch was applied to synergistic muscles to obtain greater proprioceptive stimulation. The next development occurred when it was found that an isometric (against resistance) contraction of an agonist (one muscle) followed by an isometric contraction of the antagonist (the opposing muscle) resulted in an increased response by the agonist. Spiral and diagonal movements proved even more effective.

The two methods used to produce these patterns are:

(a) *Slow reversal.* An active contraction against resistance of the agonist followed by an isotonic contraction against resistance in the antagonist without relaxation between the two. The movements are all facilitated (guided) by the therapist's hands, and the patient's actual involvement is obtained by simple commands to 'pull up' or 'push down' or 'hold' or 'relax'.

(b) *Rhythmic stabilisation.* The patient is told to contract strongly against the therapist's resistance, then to hold as an equal amount of resistance is applied alternately to the agonist and antagonist muscles by the therapist. These alternating contractions result in an increased build-up of tension in the muscle.

For example, when there is limitation of flexion of the elbow joint, the elbow is flexed to its maximum, then extension of the elbow by the triceps is carried out against the resistance supplied by the therapist. It is found that this substantially increases flexion.

Common Sports Injuries: Treatment and Recovery Time

Direct injury of the soft tissues causes bruising and contusion of the skin, pannicular tissues, muscles, and to the bony structures including that of the joints. Indirect injury results in strains, with tearing of the muscles, tendons and ligaments, and sprains, subluxations and dislocations of the joints.

In each case, the degree of injury depends on its severity and is divided into mild, moderate and severe: all must be treated by the AT Approach.

It would seem that the recovery time in all cases of direct injury coincides roughly with that of indirect injury, provided this approach is adopted. It implies urgency in treatment at every phase in which treatment time, including home treatment, occupies at least three hours daily. Long periods of rest are combined with Ice packs, Compression and Elevation (ICE – see page 102), particularly in the early stages.

DIRECT INJURY

Mild Degree. Recovery time is usually within a few days, and a further few days may be needed before the patient is completely recovered. By seven days he should be fit to return fully to his sport.

Moderate Degree. Should become symptom-free after ten days, but it is likely to be another week before the patient can return to his sport.

Severe Degree. Usually takes six to eight weeks, but if tissue necrosis (death) has occurred it may be several months before returning to full activity is possible. However, the patient must be encouraged not to give up but to carry out his routine home treatment at least twice daily, without ceasing.

The severe type may be associated with a fracture or joint instability from a ruptured ligament. These cases may be best treated in a plaster cast for three weeks, or in some cases operative interference is necessary. If in plaster, it is essential to commence isometric exercises against the resistance of the plaster immediately. If not in plaster, various forms of physiotherapy are given daily. Support is given by the Robert Jones method with wool or gamgee and bandages.

EXAMPLE

A polo player sustained a fall from his horse and, as he fell, the horse kicked him on the left side of his back in the upper lumbar region, and at the same time his saddle was forced upwards between his legs, causing a simple rupture of the urethra. This latter injury necessitated the use of an indwelling catheter for a few days. The back injury resulted in a large extravasation of blood into the tissues of the left loin, and X-rays revealed considerable displacement of his left kidney, but no fractures. On the fifth day operative evacuation of the haematoma in the left loin was made by two incisions, as the swelling appeared to be maximal at two points. Over a litre of blood was evacuated and his haemoglobin fell to sixty per cent. The wounds healed quickly, but on six occasions over the next four weeks blood-stained serum was evacuated by aspiration. Daily physiotherapy and home treatment was commenced on the seventh day, and he recovered so well that he was able to start practising polo three weeks after the original injury, and actually played in a match exactly five weeks after his accident. Treatment by the AT Approach saved him weeks of disability with complications.

If only the pannicular subcutaneous tissue is involved, recovery time may be only a few days in spite of the fact that extensive and widespread discoloration of the skin may be present even remote from the site of injury. Two types of haematoma associated with direct injury to muscles may be presented:

1. The Intermuscular Type

This type disperses quickly, especially if helped. The blood spreads through the tissues as previously mentioned, directed by the forces of gravity downwards, along the line of the blood vessels, and along the tissue planes, aided by the action of the muscles, and coming more and more to the surface. Its absorption is helped by graduated exercises, hot and cold baths or ice, ultrasound, massage and faradic contractions to all the surrounding muscles. Discoloration of the skin by blood pigments denotes the 'seeping' process into the surrounding tissues. In this process of 'seeping' the tissues become tender, and this is said to be due to the blood pigment haemosiderin.

2. The Intramuscular Type

If the amount of bruising and haematoma formation is relatively small, complete absorption takes place in a few days, helped by modified exercises and ultrasound. However, if the amount is large, total absorption may take weeks, and during this time all the complications of haematoma formation may occur. The complications of unabsorbed haematoma are:
  (a) An encysted swelling with serum in the centre.
  (b) A fibro-fatty mass in subcutaneous tissue.
  (c) A clot undergoing fatty and pigment changes.
  (d) Painful thickenings: these are situated where there is convergence of the tissue planes forming 'dead' areas or near blood vessels.
  (e) An area of myositis ossificans (bone formation in the muscle – that is, ossified haematoma), or fibrotic muscle.

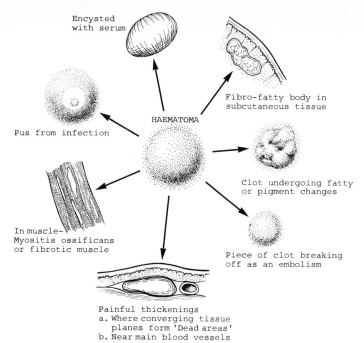

Encysted with serum

Fibro-fatty body in subcutaneous tissue

HAEMATOMA

Pus from infection

Clot undergoing fatty or pigment changes

Piece of clot breaking off as an embolism

In muscle-Myositis ossificans or fibrotic muscle

Painful thickenings
a. Where converging tissue planes form 'Dead areas'
b. Near main blood vessels

Figure 21. Complications of a large haematoma. This is the reason for immediate action to cause its removal either by the Active Therapeutic Approach or surgical evacuation.

(f) The mass becoming infected with pus formation.

(g) In the early stages when a large haematoma forms in the tissue, clotting occurs and there is the chance of an embolism spreading to the lungs. This is a complication which should always be considered, and therefore the presence of an unabsorbed haematoma in the muscles should be taken relatively seriously.

One or more of these complications have been noted in sports injuries many months after the original accident, and have accounted for recurrence or failure in healing, making return to full activity impossible until the complications have been rectified.

If the blood collection in the intramuscular type is superficial – that is, on the surface of the muscle mass such as the quadriceps – quick absorption can be stimulated by contrast baths, faradism and ultrasound, with massage to the surrounding tissues as it spreads outwards. Massage to the actual area of bruising is avoided. If absorption tends to be slow, injection into the central mass with 10 ml xylocaine one per cent, with 10 ml urea and salicylic acid and 2 ml hyalase will help to break it up, and cause it to

120

spread more rapidly. If, however, the mass is soft and fluctuant, it may be possible to aspirate its contents through a large bore needle, after anaesthetising the area with one per cent xylocaine, using 10–15 ml, or, if the blood is clotted, through a small incision, also under local anaesthetic. It is imperative to incise the deep fascia so as to allow upward seepage through the muscle fibres. Sinus forceps can be inserted through the deep fascia and muscle sheath into the substance of the haematoma, as by Hilton's method of opening an abscess.

If the haematoma mass is deep down next to bone, in the substance of a muscle such as the quadriceps, a great deal of wasted time and complications can be avoided by its operative removal under general anaesthetic through a relatively small incision in the skin and muscle substance, expressing its contents and controlling any bleeding point. Suction drainage may be essential for forty-eight hours, and graduated exercises with other forms of physical treatment are indicated. If not treated in this way, the quadriceps quickly lose their ability to stretch – that is to say, the knee loses its flexibility. Gentle, but progressive physiotherapy and home treatment should be started the day after operation, and complete recovery should have taken place in three weeks. This implies that full flexion of the knee has been restored, so that the patient can sit back on his heels.

Most orthopaedic surgeons realise the importance of early evacuation of haematoma formation in which there has been extensive bruising and contusion of the soft tissues. However, as many of these cases are seen by physicians first, valuable time is often lost. Operation on those cases in which the haematoma is near to the bone must be carried out at once or within the first few days; otherwise, if operation takes place later or when there is evidence of myositis ossificans (ossified haematoma) on the radiographs, it is too late, as the condition will be worsened by the operative procedure. If a slight shadow of calcification is seen on the radiographs, these cases require complete rest – for example, in the case of the quadriceps, in a split plaster cast for eight weeks, so as to avoid aggravation. If this period of relative masterly inactivity is not instituted, there is great danger of massive bone formation in the quadriceps, which may prevent complete flexion of the knee, and the sportsman may have to give up all forms of sport permanently. The cast is removed daily for baths and quadriceps contractions, but no flexion ones are allowed. Gentle faradic stimulation of the muscles and ultrasound, with kaolin compresses at night, help to reduce the mass without stimulating it to massive bone

121

formation. When the bone shadow has become circumscribed by radiographs, in about eight weeks, knee flexion exercises can be started.

Direct Injury to Bone

The amount of traumatic swelling will naturally vary according to the degree of injury. In a mild contusion there may be only superficial bruising of the periosteum which will absorb if treated urgently in a few days. Of course a severe direct injury may result in a transverse or comminuted (multiple) fracture.

Often a moderate-size haematoma forms subcutaneously and before it has time to spread it should be evacuated under local or a general anaesthetic. The latter gives the surgeon more freedom to do the evacuation more completely; otherwise, even using local anaesthetic the procedure can be painful. The AT Approach is essential because otherwise local thickenings occur on the bone and in the surrounding tissue.

EXAMPLE

An athlete, a detective sergeant, was kicked on the shin in the course of arresting a thief. He attended several hospitals but a year later was seen with a thickening of the shin where he had been kicked and several localised thickenings in the muscles of the calf. His treatment up to then had been inadequate. With intensive treatment, including injections to the local thickenings, he made a complete recovery in six weeks.

Direct Injury to Joints

Swelling of a joint due to haemorrhagic (bloody) or synovial (fluid) effusion may require repeated aspirations combined with physical and home treatments. Injections of xylocaine and hydrocortisone may be necessary, but should be limited to no more than six injections over six weeks.

Owing to bruising and contusion of articular cartilage, recovery may take months and will only become one-hundred-per-cent right by diligent physiotherapy and home treatment. If a piece of cartilage is broken off and locking occurs, operative interference may be necessary, and a quicker result is established. This also applies to crushing of tissues within the joint. Arthroscopy will help in making the decision whether the joint should be explored. Minor degrees may be put right in a fortnight, whereas moderate degrees take two months, and severe degrees an in-

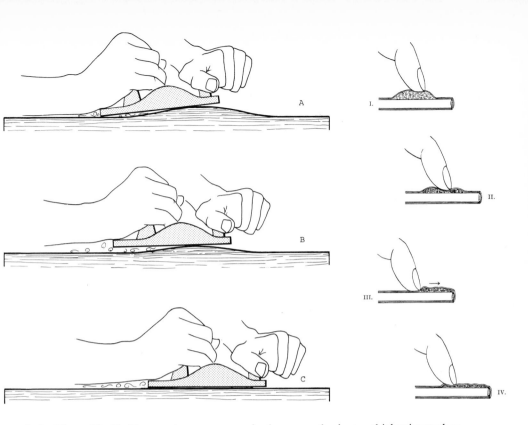

Left: Figure 22. To illustrate how a carpenter's plane smooths down a thickening such as a notch in a piece of wood (A-C). Similarly, if a thickening forms in the tissues, methods employed in the Active Therapetic Approach must gradually dissipate the thickening. Often, during the dispersal, the thickening will cause a click or clonk on movement.
Right: Figure 23. Chronic tenosynovitis, following an acute sprain or direct blow. (I) shows thickening of a tendon sheath, as the result of old injury; (II) shows that the massaging finger has broken the thickening up into fibrous nodules, one type of meton seed body; (III) shows the massage finger pushing these fibrous bodies up to the tendon sheath; (IV) shows massaging finger trapping fibrous bodies which are exquisitely tender, and breaking them up further so that they can be absorbed.

definite period. This is because if erosion of articular cartilage has occurred, regeneration of the cartilage has to take place and this may take several months.

INDIRECT INJURY: STRAINS AND TEARS OF MUSCLES AND TENDONS
In the same way these can be divided into mild, moderate and severe

123

degrees and the time incurred for complete recovery is nearly the same as for contusions and bruising of the soft tissues except where there is a complete rupture of a muscle or tendon as occurs in the tendo-Achilles at the back of the heel, three inches from its insertion.

Mild strains should be one-hundred-per-cent cured in one week and back to full activity in two weeks. Often this disability time can be limited to a few days.

Moderate strains with possible tearing of a few fibres require two weeks' intensive treatment to become symptom-free with full recovery of extensibility and contractibility, and a further two weeks' intensive training before full participation in sport is allowed. These periods of recovery can often be improved considerably by injections of xylocaine 5 mls with 10 mls of urea and salicylic acid into the area of the tear, but hydrocortisone must be avoided in tears of the weight-bearing muscles such as the tendo-Achilles.

Severe tears, amounting to rupture, may require suture, firm healing of the muscle and its tendon taking ten to twelve weeks; very careful rehabilitation is required for a further ten to twelve weeks. Return to full normal power required for vigorous exercise may take five to six months. From the end of the sixth week onwards the patient must be given a regular regime of home treatment three times daily with physiotherapy, if available, three times weekly until the twelfth week. Modified exercise such as golf and tennis may then be possible, but return to competitive athletics such as running and football may take a full six months. This applies particularly to complete rupture of the tendo-Achilles even if treated by conservative methods in a plaster of Paris cast.

TO ILLUSTRATE A MUSCLE ALERTED
It accepts a shock strain

Figure 24. Effect of shock strain on alerted and slack muscle.

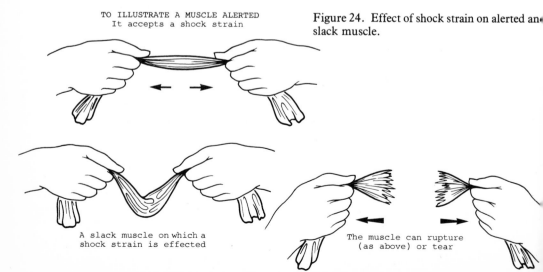

A slack muscle on which a
shock strain is effected

The muscle can rupture
(as above) or tear

Joint Strains and Sprains caused by Indirect Injury

Mild Degree. The muscles and tendons are affected by being stretched usually on one side of the joint and there is local swelling in relation to the structures with pain if they are put on the stretch. These cases should be made symptom-free usually in a few days.

Moderate Degree. The joint structures on one side of the joint are often torn, particularly the ligamentous tissues, and the soft tissue structures on the opposite side of the joint may be contused and bruised by the force of a bony structure on them. (See Figure 13, page 94.) The synovial membrane is often contused or pinched with a resulting synovial effusion or, if torn, probably a resulting haemarthrosis. By the AT Approach it is possible to make this type of case symptom-free in a fortnight and it may be another fortnight before vigorous games can be played.

Severe Degree. These are frequently associated with fractures and dislocations, or both. However, in a severely sprained joint in which there is no fracture or torn intra-articular structures, there is likely to be a large effusion, either synovial or haemorrhagic in nature. Whether medium or severe, these should be treated as follows: aspiration of synovial fluid or blood; support in a padded split plaster; isometric exercises against resistance of plaster; non-weight-bearing or non-strain exercises out of plaster after the second day; physiotherapy – ultrasound, short-wave, wax, interferential, massage and gentle manipulations; walking – partial weight-bearing in plaster with crutches or sticks for the joints of the lower extremity.

However, in some severe cases the articular cartilage is damaged or there is an internal derangement of the joint. Operative interference may be necessary because it gives a quicker result by removing contused, bruised or torn tissues. In some of these severe cases there is death of the tissues by the injury and if a conservative approach is adopted, a lengthy negative phase of recovery has to take place before the positive healing phase starts and it may be even a whole year or more before it is possible to return to full activity.

As in direct injuries to joints, the contused bruised tissues may be so damaged that they become dead tissues and will never return to normal healthy tissue. If severe, a quicker result will be achieved if they are removed by operation. However, is some cases prolonged vigorous treatment, including regular home treatment and physiotherapy, may convert the damaged tissue back to a near normal structure. This will only happen if the treatment is persevered with, relentlessly, month after month until complete regeneration has taken place. The alternative is gradual deterioration of the joint structures with the onset of osteoarthritis.

Injuries to Tendons

Injuries to the tendons of the hands and feet with the carpal, tarsal, metacarpal, metatarsal and phalangeal joint involvement, whether direct or indirect, become difficult to get one-hundred-per-cent right unless treated immediately by the AT Approach. Such cases treated in the first day by contrast baths, wax baths, ultrasound, faradism and as firm massage as possible, combined with active graduated movements, elevation and suitable support, can become symptom-free within two or three days. If left they will sometimes take at least three months or longer, or even need operative intervention before they recover.

Because in all cases it is a question of blood supply, modified activity is essential at all stages, up to the point of pain and just a little further if possible. However, if gross adhesions have formed between a tendon and its sheath, operative removal of a portion of the sheath and the freeing of the tendon completely may be necessary. Before contemplating operation in chronic tenosynovitis (inflammation of the tendon sheaths) of the tendons around the ankle, wrist and fingers, injections of xylocaine and Depomedrone should be tried on two or three occasions, followed by concentrated physiotherapy. If after one month's conservative treatment there is no improvement and gross adhesions are still present, operation is indicated. In some cases where there is a large hard swelling of the tendon and its sheath which has been present for several months, conservative treatment will almost certainly fail, and therefore immediate operation is indicated, as it will be the quickest method of promoting recovery.

Bursae

There are superficial bursal sacs interposed between the skin and bony points, and deep ones between the muscles and other bony points. These are most important structures, as they are liable to suffer changes from injury or gout, or because they are firmly attached to their deeper structures by inflammatory changes. They may also be the subject of attribution by weak muscles, causing rubbing against an underlying bony prominence. The common superficial ones are over the knee-cap (the

126

pre-patellar bursa or housemaid's knee), over the point of the elbow (olecronon bursa), and over the tuber ischii, which is called the tailor's bursa, as the tailor sits on it in his work.

Deeper ones are the ileo-psoas bursa in front of the hip joint, the gluteal bursa under the insertion of the gluteus maximus, the sub-acromial bursa under the deltoid at the shoulder.

Injury to the bursae, especially the superficial ones, will cause a synovitis or a haemorrhage, and if this takes place they become enlarged, swollen and painful. Removal of the fluid by aspiration becomes essential. This can usually be accomplished under a local anaesthetic. Short-wave, ultrasound and friction massage is necessary in most cases to absorb and break up small, gritty, granular, fibrous bodies, which form particularly in the sub-acute and chronic types. Depomedrone 2 ml with 5 ml one per cent xylocaine also helps to absorb these products, and hasten recovery. If there is a gouty diathesis this must be treated. Rarely does removal of these bursae become necessary.

In the case of the semi-membranosus bursa, and occasionally in the sub-acromial bursa, calcareous bodies form, requiring removal of the bodies and even the bursa.

Subluxation of a Joint

Ligaments may have been torn, but if after reduction a well-moulded support of the Robert Jones type (gamgee and bandages) is applied over the injured joint, isometric exercises and other forms of physiotherapy can be started at once and carried out daily.

Recovery time is two weeks to become symptom-free; four weeks for strenuous exercise. Of course, these times will depend on the subluxation becoming relatively stable. Operation is rarely required unless the sub-luxation keeps on recurring so as to make it impossible for the athlete to return to his sport. Examples of joints which may be affected are the facet joints, particularly of the lower lumbar vertebrae, the ankle joints and the acromio-clavicular (outer end of collar bone) joint.

Dislocation of a Joint

Reduction must be carried out as soon as possible and careful X-rays taken before and after reduction to ascertain whether there is an associated fracture. If the reduction is stable and there is no fracture, a plaster cast support is applied and split at the end of three weeks, but in the interval vigorous isometric exercises are carried out daily, combined, if possible, with faradic contraction of the muscles above and below the plaster. As soon as the plaster is split it is removed for daily physiotherapy and baths. A lower limb joint is allowed to bear weight partially with crutches after five weeks and fully as soon as painless movements allow.

Cases in which the joint is unstable after reduction may require immediate surgery. After operation the joint is immobilised in a plaster cast for a month, but isometric movements are started the day following surgery, and after a month, the plaster is split and the patient then treated in the same way as a stable dislocation after reduction.

Nerve Injuries

In athletes, nerves can be bruised and contused or stretched and suffer from contusion called neurapraxia (non-degenerative nerve lesion). Recovery can take anything from a few days to six months before it is complete. Electromyographic tests are helpful in prognosis.

Occasionally associated with either simple or compound fractures there may be rupture of the nerve fibres within the sheath, axonotmesis (syndrome of lesion in continuity). Signs of recovery may take six months to appear. When the nerve is completely severed as by the sharp point of a fractured bone, this is called neurotmesis (syndrome of complete interruption) and unless the ends are approximated, recovery cannot take place. Surgery is often necessary to be sure that approximation of the ends are present and the ends are sutured. The recovery rate is, on average, one inch a month and can be demonstrated by Tinel's sign. This consists of tapping the nerve and noting tingling along its course, which would be expected to be six inches below the suture line after six months.

Wynn Parry (*Journal of Bone and Joint Surgery*, 1961) has given a comprehensive survey of the importance of electro diagnosis. It studies the reaction of voluntary muscles and nerves to electrical stimuli by:
1. *Tests for nerve conduction.* Stimulation of superficial motor nerve by surface electrode and observing contraction of the muscles enervated by that nerve.
2. *Intensity duration curves* are a study of the reaction of voluntary muscles and nerves to electrical stimuli of known strength and known duration. These are graphic expressions of the excitability of neuro-muscular tissues.

128

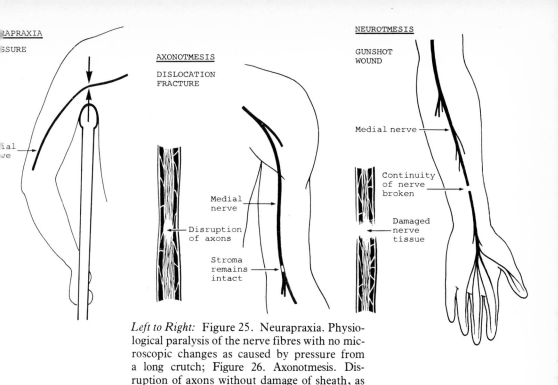

AXONOTMESIS

DISLOCATION
FRACTURE

GUNSHOT
WOUND

Medial nerve

ial
ve

Continuity
of nerve
broken

Medial
nerve

Disruption
of axons

Damaged
nerve
tissue

Stroma
remains
intact

Left to Right: Figure 25. Neurapraxia. Physiological paralysis of the nerve fibres with no microscopic changes as caused by pressure from a long crutch; Figure 26. Axonotmesis. Disruption of axons without damage of sheath, as can be caused by a dislocation or fracture; Figure 27. Neurotmesis. The continuity of the nerve is broken, as can be caused by a bullet.

The Entrapment Syndrome

It has been said that every nerve in the body can be subjected to pressure from fibrous tissue bands. The better known ones are:

1. The median nerve in the carpal tunnel.
2. The posterior tibial nerve as it enters the inner aspect of the foot.
3. The ulnar nerve as it passes behind the medial condyle of the humerus and again lower down in the vicinity of the hook of the hamate in the hand.
4. The suprascapular nerve as it passes under the suprascapular notch of the scapula.
5. The lateral cutaneous nerve of the thigh as it passes under Poupart's ligament.
6. The dorsal interosseous branch of the radial nerve as it passes under the fibrous origin of the extensor carpi radialis brevis.

In certain cases where there are only early sensory changes in a nerve

I

due to pressure, this may be relieved with injections of xylocaine one per cent 10 mls, with 2 mls of Depomedrone around the nerve at the point of pressure.

This is followed by concentrated physiotherapy.

When there is evidence of motor involvement immediate operative relief of the pressure is essential.

Fractures

Fractures are naturally more common in the sports in which there are quick movements at high speeds, as in motor-car motor-cycle, steeple-chasing and skiing events. They also occur in any type of football and, to a lesser extent, in cricket, ice hockey and any contact sports in which human bodies come together or in which falls take place. Fractures can also occur from direct blows from a fast-travelling object, such as a cricket ball, baseball or javelin.

Armstrong (*Injury in Sport*, 1964) describes five types of mechanical forces too great for bone to bear and which cause fractures:

1. A direct force at right angles to the long axis of a bone produces a transverse fracture; where a severe force from an outside agent is applied to a bone, a comminuted fracture may result.

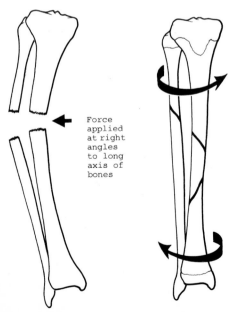

Force applied at right angles to long axis of bones

Far left: Figure 28. Effect of direct force at right angles to long axis of bones. *Left:* Figure 29. Indirect violence causing rotatory force producing oblique or spinal fracture.

2. Indirect violence causing a rotatory force resulting in an oblique fracture in relation to the long axis or usually where there are two bones – fibula and tibia (in the lower leg) – the latter bone may only be broken and the fracture is spiral.
3. Force transmitted along the bone itself resulting in a crush or compression of the bone and fracture.
4. Force transmitted through a muscle to a bone resulting in the avulsion of a piece of bone with muscle insertion.

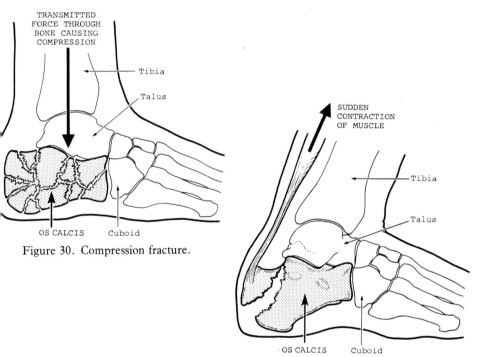

Figure 30. Compression fracture.

Figure 31. Fracture from strong muscular contraction.

5. Fatigue or stress fracture. (See overleaf.)

Fractures are also divided into simple and closed (in which the skin is not broken), or compound and open (in which the skin is broken and a sinus track runs down to the site of the fracture). In open or compound fractures, as soon as the skin has been closed and healed, the fracture becomes a simple or closed fracture. Wound toilet in fractures of this type must be carried out as soon as possible.

131

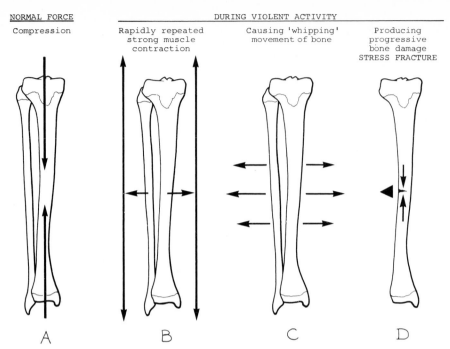

Compression | Rapidly repeated strong muscle contraction | Causing 'whipping' movement of bone | Producing progressive bone damage STRESS FRACTURE

A   B   C   D

Figure 32. How a stress fracture occurs from a whipping force in the leg bones. Normally the main force, which is the body weight, falls on a long bone, compressing it (A). During violent activity the forces produced by rapidly repeated strong contraction of the various muscle groups are added to that of gravity (B). This causes a whipping movement of the bone (C). If continued for a sufficiently long time, this movement produces progressive bone damage, known as 'stress fracture' (D). (*After Mr J. R. Armstrong, joint author of* Injury in Sport.)

Watson-Jones (1964) described three essentials in the treatment of fractures:

1. Reduction: Displacement of the fragments must be corrected and re-displacement prevented.
2. Immobilisation: The fragments must be immobilised completely, continuously and without interruption until union is firm. This applies particularly to unstable fractures.
3. Functional activity: Joints which need not be immobilised must be actively exercised but never passively stretched.

If in plaster the muscles overlying the fractured bones must be made to move by isometric exercises against the resistance of the plaster.

132

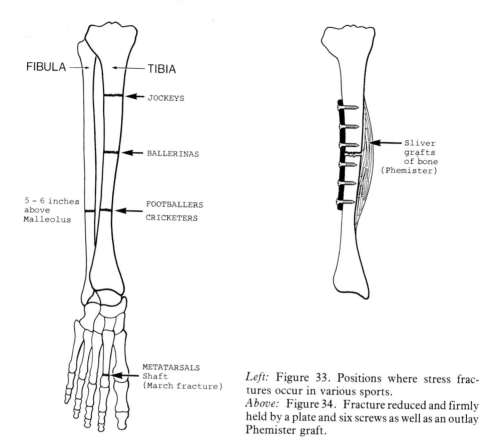

FIBULA — TIBIA

JOCKEYS

BALLERINAS

5 – 6 inches above Malleolus

FOOTBALLERS CRICKETERS

METATARSALS Shaft (March fracture)

Sliver grafts of bone (Phemister)

Left: Figure 33. Positions where stress fractures occur in various sports.
Above: Figure 34. Fracture reduced and firmly held by a plate and six screws as well as an outlay Phemister graft.

Watson-Jones described four methods of reduction and immobilisation: manipulative reduction and plaster immobilisation; manipulative reduction and continuous skin traction; manipulative reduction and skeletal traction; operative reduction and internal fixation.

Surgeons will differ in their methods of reduction and immobilisation. In some hospitals one team will carry out reductions and immobilisation in plaster, whereas another team will carry out reduction and internal fixation as by the methods of the Association for the Study of the Problems of Internal Fixation (AO). These methods of internal fixation have been perfected by famous Swiss Professors M. E. Müller, M. Allgöwer, and H. Willenegger.

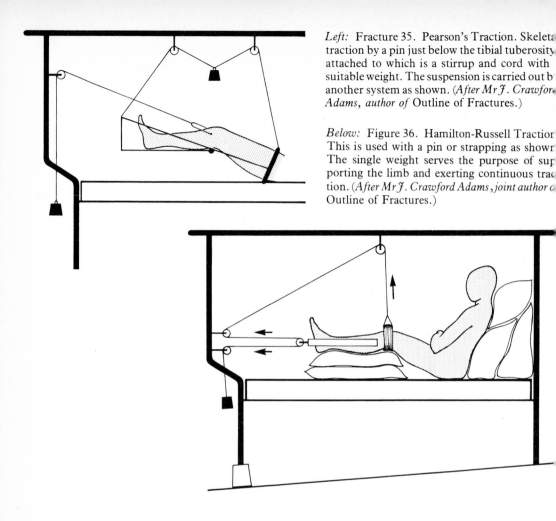

Left: Fracture 35. Pearson's Traction. Skeleta traction by a pin just below the tibial tuberosity attached to which is a stirrup and cord with suitable weight. The suspension is carried out b another system as shown. (*After Mr J. Crawfor Adams, author of* Outline of Fractures.)

Below: Figure 36. Hamilton-Russell Tractior This is used with a pin or strapping as showr The single weight serves the purpose of sup porting the limb and exerting continuous trac tion. (*After Mr J. Crawford Adams, joint author c* Outline of Fractures.)

Lucas Champonnière, a famous French surgeon during the middle of the last century, treated all fractures by the same method – with immediate movement of the muscles and joints. Of course, he should have distinguished between fractures which were stable and those which were unstable. The stable fracture, which is not displaced, may require only a plaster of Paris cast which can be split so as to allow modified movements, and physiotherapy to absorb the traumatic swellings. Early exercise of the overlying muscles of a non-straining nature quickly helps to absorb traumatic swellings, including excessive fracture haematoma and maintains muscle power.

If the fracture is impacted or there is a simple crack, exercises should

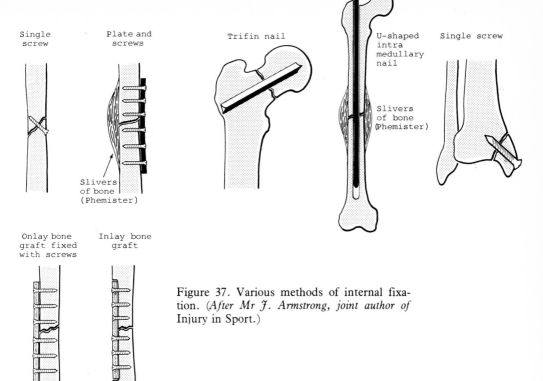

Single screw · Plate and screws · Trifin nail · U-shaped intra medullary nail · Single screw

Slivers of bone (Phemister)

Slivers of bone (Phemister)

Onlay bone graft fixed with screws · Inlay bone graft

Figure 37. Various methods of internal fixation. (*After Mr J. Armstrong, joint author of* Injury in Sport.)

take place from the onset, the fracture supported by gamgee and crêpe bandage, or rested and supported in a split plaster which can easily be removed. Exercises which can be carried out isometrically against the resistance of the plaster prevent pooling of venous blood, and encourage the circulation of arterial blood, which promotes callus formation. It has been our practice to stimulate the muscles through windows cut in the plaster by the labile faradic method. In delayed union the modern method is employed of stimulating the fractured ends by the negative electrode of a direct current machine.

Faradic stimulation of the muscles is a more active way of encouraging callus formation, by pulling on the periosteal attachments of the muscles around the fracture site. Care should be taken not to overstimulate these attachments in relation to joints, especially the elbow and knee, as this may cause excessive bone formation. However, this complication is academic rather than real.

135

FATIGUE OR STRESS FRACTURES

These were originally called 'March fractures' because they were common in young soldiers of both world wars. It has been said that any bone in the body can be subject to a 'fatigue' or 'stress' fracture. There is a preliminary phase in which there is pain and swelling of the soft tissue over the site where the fracture later occurs.

Armstrong's explanation is probably the best, which is that of a whipping force affecting the bone at the point of stress (Figure 32, page 132). However, in the sportsman it is most commonly in the metatarsal bones (the front transverse arch), and to a lesser extent in the tibia at various levels (see Figure 33, page 133), and the fibula. Poor posture and the wrong execution of actions usually are a constant factor. In the early stages there may be no X-ray changes, but if the condition is treated by the AT Approach – that is, rest from strain, attention to correct posture, home treatment and physiotherapy – radiographic changes with evidence of fracture may be averted. In some cases, in the early stages, before X-rays show a fracture, there is pain and swelling and a sudden extra strain, such as occurs during jumping, will produce sharp pain with a tender area and swelling, and by then the radiographic films will show a fatigue fracture.

Shin soreness is often a precursor of a stress or fatigue fracture of the tibia. These cases should be taken seriously, and treated as suggested. Sometimes, with the aid of local injections of xylocaine, urea and salicylic acid, they can be checked in three weeks and, provided the patient adopts correct posture and execution of movements, the condition is arrested and does not recur.

Many surgeons, particularly in the United States of America and England, still prefer the conservative approach in the treatment of fractures – that is to say, they do not believe in internal fixation except under exceptional circumstances. At an International Orthopaedic Meeting, Allgöwer and Müller read a paper on the results of over five hundred cases of fracture of the tibia and fibula which, by their method of internal fixation, were fully rehabilitated in 132 days. Two American Army orthopaedic surgeons read a similar paper on five hundred cases of tibia and fibula treated by conservative reduction held in plaster of Paris, and their cases also took 132 days to be completely rehabilitated. They were prepared to accept up to half-an-inch shortening, whereas by the Swiss Compression System alignment was perfect, and there was no shortening. However, a second operation is necessary under the latter method, and the chance of infection by open reduction, plating and screwing does occur. In practically every case both methods of treatment eventually produced satisfactory results.

In Switzerland special plates and screws are used for each type of fracture treated by their method. In some cases of femoral fractures two plates and screws are sometimes considered necessary.

Küntscher popularised the intramedullary nailing of fractures, and in athletes, if a fracture required internal fixation, this method would seem to be the least traumatic. At the same time, or two weeks later, Phemister bone slivers can be placed around the fracture site to ensure early consolidation.

The Swiss Compression System gives beautiful fixation of fractures in exact anatomical position, but in all cases it is advised that the plate and screws should be removed after consolidation has taken place – that is to say, after about eighteen months at a convenient time. This means that the sportsman, if he is a professional, has to be off his job for a second period. Apart from that, the screw holes are always in a place where potential stress fractures can occur. In long bones, therefore, fixation by intramedullary nailing combined with Phemister grafting usually allows return to full activity in three months, without the need necessarily for a second operation, unless the nail gives trouble.

The concomitant injuries of the soft tissues in the neighbourhood of the fracture, as well as mobility in the joints above and below, must always be considered. For example, Lester Lowe reported two cases in which there had been severe fractures of the tibial plateau near the knee joint; one was compounded with a dirty wound, and the other comminuted with a certain amount of disturbance of the tibial plateau. The former was treated conservatively by traction. Movements of the knee were encouraged, and with proper treatment of the skin wound, union and a mobile knee resulted quickly. The other tibial fracture was treated with reconstruction of the tibial plateau with plates and screws, resulting in a stiff knee and not nearly such a good result.

For years we have employed Perkins' method of treating fractures around joints, especially the knee and elbow, with traction in as full extension as possible. Extension either by skin traction or skeletal traction is applied, and very gentle knee and elbow movements started immediately. Often severely comminuted fractures fall into place. Muscle wasting is prevented by the exercises, and the muscles are stimulated by faradism for fifteen minutes daily if necessary. Full extension is maintained and flexion exercises carried out against the resistance of the weight extension from the beginning. Full movement can be eighty per cent in eight weeks and one hundred per cent in four months, when full activity can be commenced. Often fractures around the elbow and knee are treated in a plaster cast for six weeks with poor results, and extremes of flexion and extension never return to normal.

The protagonists of the Swiss Compression System claim that many cases of fractures in the vicinity of a joint which has been treated by their method avoid osteoarthritic changes in the surrounding joints, because the joints are able to be used actively at an early stage. However, if fractures near to joints are gradually reduced by traction with active exercises and daily sessions of faradism from the beginning, good function is obtained without the use of a great deal of metal.

FRACTURES OF THE LOWER EXTREMITY

It is good practice to get these fractures moving as soon as possible. Isometric exercises are carried out against the resistance of the plaster, aided if necessary by faradic stimulation of the muscles through windows in the plaster.

In the lower extremity, as soon as the fracture is stable after about three or four weeks, a walking plaster is applied, and if necessary this can be constructed so as to take counter-pressure against the ischial tuberosity in a long plaster. This incorporates a Thomas's splint which has had the top ring removed.

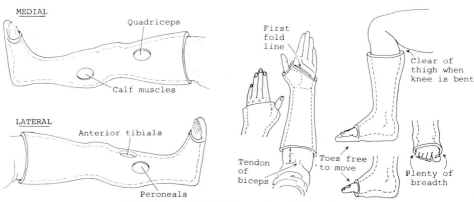

138

Left: Figure 38. Windows through the plaster of Paris at motor points to enable the administration of surging faradism. *Right:* Figure 39. Plaster for Colles' and Potts' fractures. Isometrics must be carried out regularly against the resistance of the plaster.

In other cases which do not require careful supervision, the ordinary above-knee plaster cast is split, but not bi-valved, as soon as possible, to allow free non-weight-bearing and non-straining exercises, with physiotherapy and exercises in baths and swimming pools. One-hundred-per-cent function as early as possible is a goal at which to aim, and this can only be done by obtaining a full range of movement in all the joints associated with the fracture. This means that in the case of a fracture in one of the extremities, each joint in that extremity, right up to its fixation to the spine, has to be exercised, and in the case of a spinal fracture there must be a full range of movement in all the spinal joints.

Sarmiento of Florida has devised a special walking-shoe which he incorporates into a walking-plaster. In the case of tibial and fibular fractures, reduction producing satisfactory alignment is carried out at once and maintained for three weeks, until the fractures are stable. He accepts up to $\frac{1}{2}$-in. shortening as satisfactory.

As soon as the fracture is stable he applies a walking-plaster, the upper part of the plaster taking pressure along the lower border of the patella and the ligamentum patellae. The bottom half of the plaster is taken down to about 6 in. above the ankle joint, and into this he incorporates metal uprights which fasten below on to the walking-shoe. He encourages weight-bearing walking after about three weeks, and reckons that union is firm by the tenth to twelfth week.

Many types of simple stable fractures can be made symptom-free quickly and, provided the fractured ends are protected and supported, in certain types of fracture the sportsman will be able to return to his sport quickly.

TRANSVERSE FRACTURES

These fractures in long bones and even in the metacarpals are sometimes slow in consolidating. Therefore, in sportsmen, especially professionals, internal fixation in the long bones with an intramedullary nail, reinforced by Phemister sliver grafts, is often indicated. This applies to fractures of the femur, tibia and fibula, humerus, ulna and radius. In the metacarpals, and in some cases, transverse fractures of the carpal scaphoid, fixation by screws, pins and grafting is indicated.

Fritz Koenig, the German surgeon, Elie and Alvin Lambart of Belgium, Lane of England and Scudder of the United States were pioneers in the treatment of fractures by internal fixation. This method was started at the beginning of this century. Their methods were improved on by the originators of the Compression System which was started in Switzerland in the 1950s.

TO SUMMARISE

When possible, the conventional, conservative methods are employed in fractures, but they must be supplemented because the need for urgency in the healing time is very important. This is accomplished by exercises at all times from the beginning, which means, if the fractured bones are in plaster, isometric exercises several times daily. Faradism through windows can be helpful. If internal fixation is necessary, a Küntscher Nail with Phemister grafting should be considered if feasible.

Some comminuted, displaced fractures around a joint may require internal fixation by the Swiss Compression System, but Willenegger himself stresses the importance of exact reduction and fixation, or the results are poor. However, in fractures around the joints it has been found that traction in extension with active movements of the muscles, and giving faradic stimulation of the muscles once daily for fifteen minutes, often allows orientation of the comminuted pieces into exact position. At the same time as traction is carried out, active flexor and extension exercises are commenced from the beginning, so that in six weeks when the healing of the fracture is firm, joint movements are almost full. If fractures around the elbow and knee are immobilised in plaster casts, they are particularly notorious for finishing stiff and painful with loss of movement. This is prevented to a large extent by the traction and activity method. George Perkins at St Thomas's Hospital was teaching this fifty years ago.

The Lower Extremity

Complete one-hundred-per-cent movement in all the joints of the lower extremity must be present for there to be full movement in each joint separately. Contraction and shortening of muscles and ligaments around the knee joint will not only influence the movements of the knee, but can affect those of the ankle and foot as well as those of the hip and low back.

Therefore in treating any joint of the lower extremity, it is essential to stress that exercises must be carried out for every joint of the lower extremity from the toes to the loin.

THE ANKLE AND FOOT (BASIC ANATOMY)

There are thirty-two separate joints associated with the ankle and foot with twenty-four synovial cavities. Each one can suffer injury, both direct and indirect, and are as follows:

1. The ankle joint formed by the lower articular surface of the tibia and the two malleoli above with the upper surface of the talus. It is a modified ginglymus or hinge joint allowing dorsiflexion 20° and plantarflexion 50°. There may be very slight involuntary joint-play movements between the talus and the tibia in a forward and backward direction 2–3°. Side movements of the talus on the tibia are very slight – 1–2° and depend on the strength of the ligaments.

2. The inferior tibio-fibular joint is included in the ankle joint, as the

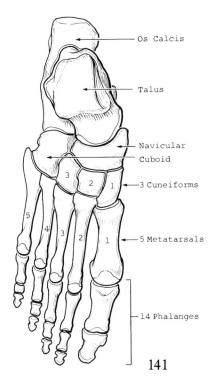

Os Calcis

Talus

Navicular

Cuboid

3 Cuneiforms

5 Metatarsals

14 Phalanges

Below: Figure 40. The right ankle and foot from the outer side. *Right:* Figure 41. The tarsal, metatarsal and phalangeal bones (top view).

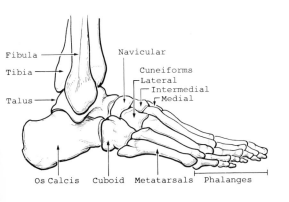

Fibula
Tibia
Talus

Navicular
Cuneiforms
Lateral
Intermedial
Medial

Os Calcis   Cuboid   Metatarsals   Phalanges

141

inferior tibio-fibular ligament makes up some of the articular surface of the ankle joint itself. It is usually a syndemosis joint, but sometimes a small pocket of synovial membrane extends from the ankle joint between the two bones. A slight gliding movement in a forward and backward direction is permitted.

3. The posterior talo-calcaneal joint is a plane joint, allowing a little antero-posterior gliding and lateral tilting (inversion 5°, and eversion 5°). This constitutes the hind foot.

4. Talo-calcaneonavicular joint is a restricted ball and socket joint and allows a combination of gliding and rotation, inversion 33°, eversion 18°.

5. Calcaneo-cuboid joint is saddle-shaped with gliding and rotation movements. This and the previous joint form the proximal mid-tarsal or transverse tarsal joints of Lisfrane and the bones of the foot distal to these joints form the forefoot in distinction to the hind foot (posterior talo-calcaneal joint).

6–8. The cuneo-navicular plane joints, allowing slight gliding movements.

9. The cubo-navicular plane joint is not constant.

10–11. The intercuneiform joints between the medial and intermediate cuneiforms and the intermediate and lateral cuneiform.

12. The tarso-metatarsal joints, all allowing slight gliding – the joints of Chopart.

13. Medial cuneo – first metatarsal.

14. The joint between the second metatarsal dovetailed between the medial and lateral cuneiforms, articulating at its base anteriorly with the intermediate cuneiform.

15. The joint between the third metatarsal and the lateral cuneiform.

16. The joint between the fourth metatarsal and the lateral cuneiform.

17–18. There may be small synovial cavities at the bases of the second and third, and third and fourth and the fourth and fifth metatarsals.

19–23. These five metatarso-phalangeal condyloid joints allow flexion, extension, adduction, abduction and circumduction and a certain amount of joint play movement of the metatarsal heads on the base of the proximal phalanges.

24–32. The big toes have only one interphalangeal joint, whereas the other four toes have two. They are hinge joints allowing flexion and extension with a certain amount of play movements between the head and base on the contiguous phalanges.

142

Injuries in the Lower Extremity

INJURIES TO THE ANKLE

Strains and sprains are divided into adduction inversion injuries and abduction eversion injuries. These can be mild, moderate or severe, according to the severity of the injury.

Adduction Inversion

This is the common sprained ankle. The foot twists inwards, causing tearing of the lateral ligamentous structures. The head of the talus is forced directly inwards on to the deep surface of the spring ligament and onto the inner and inferior aspects of the mid-tarsal joints, causing contusion of these structures.

If the sportsman is simply walking along and the foot is placed on uneven ground and the ankle turns over, the front fibres of the lateral collateral ligament are stretched and a few may tear. This degree can usually recover in a few days, which allows return to games within a week. However, if the patient is running and the foot ricks, the talus and the foot are twisted inwards and become fixed on the ground. This allows the lower articular surface of the tibia to skate forwards on the underlying talus. As this surface of the talus is narrower behind and wider in front, the tibia becomes jammed forwards and constitutes a definite subluxation. To reduce the subluxation the heel is pulled downwards and forwards with one hand, exerting some traction as well, and the tibia at the ankle joint pushed backwards with the other hand, when a 'clonk' denoting reduction of the subluxation is felt. The patient is conscious of immediate relief.

INJURIES TO THE POSTERIOR PART OF THE LATERAL (TALO-FIBULAR) LIGAMENT

Strains or tears of this ligament cause pain and stiffness and inability to hit a football with the instep. If, after one month, the patient is not symptom-free, manipulative stretching under general anaesthetic is often necessary.

Xylocaine one per cent in 5 ml with 1 ml of Depomedrone 40 mg is given to the area of the ligament after the manipulation. The essential movements in the manipulation are to pull the heel inwards and at the same time move the forefoot outwards so as to put the ligament on full stretch.

In the severe type of sprained ankle there may be rupture of the lateral ligament with a fracture of the outer surface of the talus and operative reconstruction of the ligament and adjustment of any bony displacement may be the quickest method to promote recovery. Sometimes the fractures of the talus on its outer side are missed unless oblique views are taken at X-ray.

EXAMPLE OF MEDIUM-TO-SEVERE SPRAINED ANKLE

An international football player sprained his right ankle on a Saturday. The ankle and foot were swollen and extremely painful, especially over the lateral collateral ligament, and when seen two days later he could not put his foot to the ground and had suffered two sleepless nights. X-rays in three planes revealed no fracture or diastasis (separation of the tibia and fibula bones), but as well as the extensive swelling of the whole foot, ankle and lower leg, there was evidence of fluid in the ankle joint by the appearance of a bulge in front of the tendo-Achilles on both sides. He was immediately put into a split plaster of Paris cast and given crutches. Treatment was started immediately and given twice daily. He also received exact instructions about home treatment to be performed three times daily. Treatment consisted of a local injection of 5 ml of one per cent xylocaine and 1 ml of hydrocortisone in the outer strained ligament, wax baths, short-wave, ultrasound and faradic stimulation of all muscles by the labile method. On the Friday, six days after the accident, he began weight-bearing and the ankle movement rapidly returned to normal so that by the following Tuesday, ten days after the injury, he started training and was able to pass a strenuous training test on the Friday,

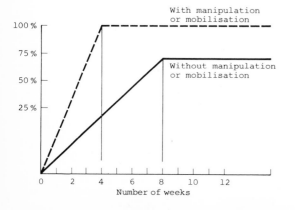

Figure 42. To demonstrate how manipulative and mobilising methods can make a joint such as the ankle one-hundred-per-cent fit in four weeks, against one in which these methods are not included in physiotherapy, and in which recovery never takes place until manipulation under an anaesthetic is carried out.

thirteen days after the injury. He was able to captain his side in a cup final exactly two weeks from the date of the injury. He stated that a few years previously he had sustained a similar injury to the left ankle but to a lesser degree and twelve weeks after injury this one had not recovered as well as the right one did in two weeks. This is a good example of the immediate application of the AT Approach firstly to absorb traumatic effusion, secondly to allow good healing and restoration of function.

Abduction Eversion

There is a tendency in severe sprains to cause a diastasis of the inferior tibio-fibular joint. If present, firm support in a complete plaster cast for two weeks may be indicated. No weight-bearing is allowed; isometric exercises against the resistance of the plaster and faradism through windows in the plaster should be considered. After two weeks, modified weight-bearing is allowed, still continuing with the isometric exercises and faradism. After four weeks the plaster is split and exercises to the ankle and foot without weight-bearing are started. This is combined with physiotherapy (short-wave, faradism, wax, ultrasound and gentle manipulative movements). After the treatment the split plaster is reapplied for walking until the ankle has active painfree movements without weight-bearing. As soon as weight-bearing in the plaster is relatively painless, which is usually about a further four weeks, the patient is allowed out of plaster with a firm bandage support. Active Alerted Posture is stressed with regards to the ankle and foot – that is to say, with the weight on the outside of the foot, rolling forwards on to the little toe and finally the big toe. When shoes or boots are allowed, an inner $\frac{3}{8}$ in. wedge placed on the heel and tread may be advisable.

THE UNSTABLE ANKLE
Due to injuries of the lateral ligament and subsequent incomplete healing, tilting of the talus out of the ankle mortice occurs and in some cases becomes so frequent as to make playing major sports impossible. In some cases the lateral ligament can be strengthened with concentrated exercises, especially eversion exercises against resistance, and this is best carried out by crossing the legs and everting and inverting each ankle against resistance of the opposite ankle. These exercises can be carried out frequently during the day, while watching television or at other times. Added to this, the ankle should be firmly strapped in eversion during

sporting activities and the sole of the shoe or boot floated out $\frac{3}{8}$ in. on the heel and tread on the outer side. This has the effect of giving a firmer and wider base to the ankle and foot and helps to prevent the ankle frequently ricking over.

Occasionally, in spite of all forms of treatment, a severe ankle injury will not respond to treatment. The talus is often found to tilt out of its mortice and re-routing of the peroneus brevis must be performed to prevent ankle instability. Sometimes there is a persistent tibio-fibular diastasis (separation) at the ankle joint. Often the patient knows nothing of Active Alerted Posture and in his everyday use of the ankle is throwing a constant strain on an already damaged ankle.

There may be persistent wasting of the foot and calf muscles so that proper muscular control of the ankle is absent. If the bony structures of the ankle have been severely bruised and contused in the original injury, recovery will not take place until all the products of bruising and contusion have been absorbed. This can only happen relatively quickly by persevering with the AT Approach until recovery takes place. In the older sportsman an early osteoarthritic process may begin to appear because the epichondrium of the articular surfaces has become involved. If this has happened the joint structures will tend to swell and become tender with exercise. However, if the sportsman is young enough and perseveres, recovery will take place slowly with increasing ability to take exercise. If these procedures are not successful, operative reinforcement of the lateral ligament should be considered, employing the Watson–Jones method of transferring the peroneus brevis through a tunnel in the lateral malleolus.

FOOTBALLER'S ANKLE
This sub-acute or chronic condition is fairly common in the seasoned footballer. It is due to constant strain on the anterior lower attachment of the capsule into the region of the neck of the talus and is caused by constant kicking of a football in the plantar-flexed position. A small fragment of bone or periosteal reaction will cause the formation of a bony bump over which the overlying capsule and tendons pass with recurrence of friction and the formation of a synovial tuft or tenovaginitis on the overlying tendons. In moderate cases, local injections of xylocaine and Depomedrone with a few physiotherapy treatments, (wax, massage and ultrasound) may produce a symptom-free state; often operative removal of the bony bump as a long-term cure is necessary.

146

Contusion Sprains of the Foot

If severe, this may require multiple small incisions to evacuate oedema and haematoma. A split plaster of Paris cast should be applied and removed for frequent contrast bathing, physiotherapy and non weight-bearing exercises. The points of incision may have to be opened up frequently to let out traumatic fluid.

Fractures of the Metatarsal Bones of the Foot

If the injury has been severe, there is often extensive bruising and contusion of the soft tissues of the foot and ankle. Protection and support with relief of weight-bearing by the use of crutches is essential.

EXAMPLE 1

A flat-race jockey fractured the neck of the fifth metatarsal of his left foot but the main injury was severe bruising and contusion of the soft tissues of the ankle and foot. These were treated by the AT Approach and he was able to race in three days. Fractures of the styloid process of the fifth metatarsal can be treated in the same way.

EXAMPLE 2

An international sportsman, who was also an actor and had to carry out a great deal of dancing in his act, sustained a similar undisplaced fracture. His ankle and foot were swollen and so painful thirty-six hours later that it was impossible for him to take any weight at all on his injured foot. However, in a further forty-eight hours he was able, by the AT Approach to perform in a complete rehearsal. Obviously the foot and ankle were well supported.

EXAMPLE 3

A steeplechase jockey sustained a fracture of the body of the os calcis with some outward displacement of the lateral fragment. However, there was no involvement of the subtaloid joint (below the ankle), but the important factor was that at the same time as the injury he had sustained a severe sprain and contusion of the ankle, mid-tarsal and forefoot joints. It was impossible for him to take any weight. He was treated in a plaster cast, which was split two days after injury, and started on physiotherapy and

147

home treatment. On the fifth day he was able to take modified weight on the ankle and foot in the cast with the help of elbow crutches, and was able to race in three weeks with protection and support to the ankle and foot with felt and bandages. As the fracture did not involve the subtaloid joint, this was possible in a jockey, as only modified weight-bearing was required, but would have been impossible in those cases in which full weight-bearing was required on the os calcis and foot. However, in this case the foot and ankle were completely symptom-free, with full movement and muscle power in a further three weeks, and all kinds of sport could have been carried out in twelve weeks.

The late Kenneth Pridie used to treat painful soles of feet resulting from severe fractures of the os calcis by removal of the os calcis. He demonstrated six cases at the Royal Society of Medicine: six policemen who were able to jump from the platform to the floor, a distance of four feet, without any pain or disability after removal of the os calcis. Somebody asked him what the patient stood on, and he replied 'On his feet, you fool!'

INJURIES TO THE SOFT TISSUE STRUCTURES BELOW THE KNEE AND ABOVE THE ANKLE

These occur as:

1. *Injuries to the components of the tendo-Achilles and injuries to the tendo-Achilles itself.* These injuries are often due to a quick contraction of the calf muscles. Fibres of the gastrocnemius or soleus or both, are torn, especially if the action has started with the feet in a flat footed position. Previously it was thought that the plantaris was involved; usually this muscle is found to escape injury.

The tendo-Achilles has a false sheath which is a thickening of the fascia over the tendon at about $3\frac{1}{2}$ in. from its insertion downwards. Occasionally a true sheath exists, with a synovial membrane. However, strains of the tendon and its covering are sometimes extremely difficult to make symptom-free quickly. Gout should be excluded. Butacote helps. Injections at weekly intervals of 10 ml one per cent xylocaine with 10 mls of urea and salicylic acid are spread around the tendon and ultrasound and friction massage given. In spite of some opinion, faradism by the labile method helps to separate the tendon from its sheath and even kaolin poultices are helpful. Treatment must include contrast baths and gradu-

148

ated exercises with attention to correct ankle and foot posture because often strains from bad posture are the cause of the condition. Treated in this way chronic resistant cases are better in a month.

Hydrocortisone must be avoided in tears of the weight-bearing muscles such as the tendo-Achilles, gastrocnemius and soleus as it may precipitate further tears or ruptures of the muscle or tendon.

Recently, recurrent cases of tendo-Achilles tendonitis have been treated by linear incisions in its sheath and tendon. The late Keon Cohen described how a small focus of granulation tissue similar to that of an osteoid osteoma in bone was found in the substance of the tendon. Removal of this restored full function. An example of this was seen in a woman Olympic gold medallist. She had had two injections of hydrocortisone into the tendon with subsequent small tears on each occasion. At operation the sheath was found firmly bound to the tendon and had to be separated carefully owing to dense adhesion formation from the tears. Three linear incisions were made vertically in the tendon and, as great strength was required, the tendon palmaris longus (front of left wrist) from the left wrist was grafted over the tendon. She made an excellent full recovery in the record time of six weeks.

Severe tears, amounting to rupture, require suturing and good firm healing will not return to normal within ten to twelve weeks. As all sportsmen require great power in their tendo-Achilles, the tendon must be strengthened with a fascial graft from the thigh or by employing the left palmaris longus in a right-handed patient. Some surgeons use the plantaris.

EXAMPLE

An international hurdler and cricketer had the torn tendon reinforced with a strip of fascia lata and was able to perform equally well after the operation as he had prior to injury.

Very careful rehabilitation is required for a further ten to twelve weeks. From the end of the sixth week onwards the patient must be given a regular regime of home treatment three times daily which has to be followed up with physiotherapy three times weekly until the twelfth week. Modified exercise such as golf or tennis may then be possible, but return to competitive sports such as running and football may take a full six months. This applies particularly to rupture of the tendo-Achilles.

2. Anterior tibial compartment syndrome. This syndrome occurs in long-distance cyclists, walkers or runners and sometimes an emergency operation has to be performed. It may also occur if there has been extensive bleeding into the anterior tibial compartment caused by a severe kick. The blood supply to the muscles of the anterior tibial compartment is at risk because of oedema of the tissues and the fact that the anterior sheath of the muscles is so thick that expansion is not possible. Relief of the pressure on the vascular structures is paramount, otherwise the muscles and tendons may undergo ischaemic necrosis as in Volkmann's ischaemia of the forearm muscles. Splitting up of the fibrous sheath of the anterior tibial compartment is all that is required and this can be carried out by a small incision top and bottom using a fasciotomy knife. Following this operation it is essential that the sportsman understands correct ankle and foot posture.

EXAMPLE

Two long-distance walkers who had undergone this operation were seen with persistent symptoms confined to the posterior part of the subcutaneous border of the tibia where the calf muscles take their origin. With attention to correct ankle and foot posture they lost their symptoms in a month. These cases often lead to shin soreness and possible stress fractures. It is conceivable that if they had learned the benefit from Active Alerted Posture neither the anterior compartment syndrome nor the subsequent shin soreness would have happened.

3. *Loss of movement in the superior and inferior tibio-fibular joints*. As a result of sprains to the knee and ankle joints these two joints are liable to injury. If they are not treated, subsequent limitation of their normal movement in a backward and forward direction becomes inevitable. Signs and symptoms are tenderness and soreness of the tissue over and around the joints with a sciatic neuritis along the lateral popliteal nerve, either on the outer side of the leg below the neck of the fibula, or down the outer side of the foot. Manipulations and physiotherapy usually restore the loss of mobility quickly. If not, one or two injections of xylocaine and Depomedrone may be necessary as well.

THE KNEE JOINT

The knee joint is a ginglymus hinge joint composed of the patello-femoral joint and two tibio-femoral compartments, the medical tibio-femoral and the lateral tibio-femoral. The pivot of movement between femoral con-

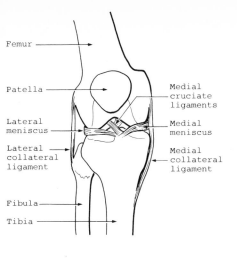

Figure 43. The right knee (front view).

Labels for Figure 43:
Femur
Patella
Lateral meniscus
Lateral collateral ligament
Fibula
Tibia
Medial cruciate ligaments
Medial meniscus
Medial collateral ligament

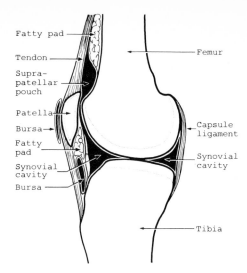

Figure 44. The right knee (inner side view).

Labels for Figure 44:
Fatty pad
Tendon
Supra-patellar pouch
Patella
Bursa
Fatty pad
Synovial cavity
Bursa
Femur
Capsule ligament
Synovial cavity
Tibia

dyles varies in flexion and extension, being posterior in flexion and more anterior in extension. The tibia also rotates medially on the femur in flexion, and from its position in full flexion, laterally in extension. This accounts for the rotating figure-of-eight movement, which can be damaging to the meniscii, which are firmly attached to the tibia at both ends. The total amount of movement from full extension, which is 0°, to full flexion is to 135° and limitation of movement is measured in relation to these amounts. If the patient has a genu recurvatum he extends past 0° to 10–15°.

In a stable joint the strong capsule is reinforced by ligaments, both the medial and the lateral collateral ligaments as well as the anterior and posterior cruciates. The latter allow a minimal amount of forward gliding of the femur on the tibia. This is described as the skating movement forwards when the weight is on the foot. Some tilting of the tibia on the femur takes place, both medially (inwards) and laterally (outwards) when the knee is relaxed. Both forward gliding and tilting are accessory to joint-play forward movements, and are present to a small degree.

In flexion and extension the patella moves downwards and upwards on its corresponding femoral surface. In a 'tight hip', the quadriceps and its attachment to the patella are short and contracted. This can cause excessive friction on the patello-femoral surface, and predispose to degenera-

151

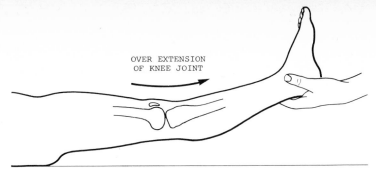

OVER EXTENSION
OF KNEE JOINT

Figure 45. Genu recurvatum. This type of knee should be given a heel raise, and it is more liable to injury than normal.

tive changes or even subluxation or dislocation of the patella.

Smillie points out in *Injuries of the Knee Joint* that certain differences in the bony construction of the knee joint predispose to injuries and conditions of stress. They are: a high patella; flat, transverse tibial condyles; genu recurvatum; lateral attachment of the ligamentum patellae.

All of these conditions can lead to changes in the pads of fat, a tendency to chondromalacia patellae or a painful swollen knee. As stated before, they are also associated with a tight hip joint, that is, one in which there is limitation of inward (internal) rotation of the hip at 90° flexion, and also limitation of the thigh with the heel on the opposite knee cap, which is the 'tailor' position.

INJURIES AND CONSEQUENT PATHOLOGICAL CONDITIONS COMMON TO THE KNEE JOINT

1. Sprained knee. The signs and symptoms may be acute, sub-acute or chronic, according to the cause are considered under the following headings. The degree of injury may be mild, moderate or severe.
2. Medial collateral ligament strain, tear or rupture.
3. Meniscus injuries.
4. Enlargement of the fatty pads.
5. Chondromalacia patellae and osteochondritis of the femoral condyles.
6. General joint laxity: the unstable knee.
7. Lateral pivot shift: derangement of the lateral tibio-femoral compartment.
8. Derangement of the medial tibio-femoral compartment in the older sportsman.

It is estimated that arthrography gives ninety-two-per-cent correct

152

clues to diagnosis, whereas arthroscopy adds another six per cent. No doubt in the future arthrography and arthroscopy will be employed in cases which are not straightforward.

Many of the older orthopaedists consider that with their many years of experience in examining and palpating knees they are able to do without these two more modern aids to diagnosis. However, in certain cases an arthrogram will help the diagnosis which, if necessary, can be doubly confirmed by arthroscopy. This procedure is carried out through a small incision, and the joint inspected in each of its compartments. The joint can be thoroughly irrigated, which also allows the evacuation of blood, joint debris and even small loose pieces of cartilage. If this is sufficient, joint inspection through a normal incision may not be necessary.

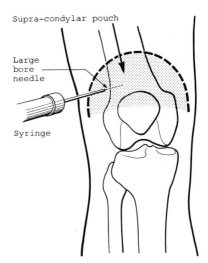

Figure 46. Aspiration of right knee.

1. Sprained Knee

The mild type should always be treated vigorously and will often be made symptom-free in a few days. In moderate and severe degrees there is often an effusion, either synovial or haemorrhagic. Removal of the fluid by aspiration is essential, especially if it is haemorrhagic, and this may have to be repeated several times. Following aspiration, hydrocortisone is not instilled into the joint if the effusion is haemorrhagic, but otherwise four injections at weekly intervals are given if necessay.

Many orthopaedic surgeons consider hydrocortisone by injection to be wrong, because it causes rapid degeneration and disintegration of the joint cartilage. A great deal depends on the positive active approach after the

153

injection as to whether the tissues heal rapidly or undergo degenerative changes. Obviously, in a frail individual hydrocortisone injections must be given cautiously.

All cases require support, modified weight-bearing activity in the early stages using sticks or crutches. Home treatment and physiotherapy is stressed. It is in the severe cases with no X-ray evidence of fracture that radiography or arthrography may be helpful to ascertain damage to the meniscii, the surfaces of the cartilage and ligamentum laxity.

If the sprained knee has been allowed to become chronic, adhesions may have formed with limitation of movement. In some cases it is best to give physiotherapy for a few days, including gentle manipulation and concentrated home treatment before considering breaking down adhesions to restore full movements. After manipulation under an anaesthetic further physiotherapy and home treatment will probably be necessary.

2(a). Medial Collateral Ligament Strain or Tear

Strain or tear of this ligament is caused by the player's foot twisting or slipping outwards, throwing a strain on the inner side of the knee, or by another player hitting the injured player a blow on the outer side of the knee. In both types of injury the medial collateral ligament is involved and, if it is associated with a twisting injury as well, the medial meniscus and the anterior cruciate ligament may be damaged, making up Don O'Donoghue's Triad.

However, in skiing the injury usually involves only the medial collateral ligament, although the other articular structures may be contused, both in the inner and outer compartments. In the pure skiing injuries in which the medial collateral ligament is injured, involvement of the medial meniscus is rare. Most of these medial collateral ligament injuries are difficult to cure quickly and often lead to a great deal of disability. There are conflicting views as to the right method of treatment. If seen several hours after injury, the overlying muscles strapping the inner, medial and posterior part of the knee have gone into spasm and flexed the knee 5–10°. This limitation of full extension can quickly simulate the symptoms of an injury of the medial meniscus. Often there is little or no effusion into the joint, but there is always an exquisitely tender point along the line of the medial collateral ligament, usually at its upper attachment.

When an abduction is thrown on the lower leg and the knee opens up more than 20° on its inner side, there is obvious marked instability of the

154

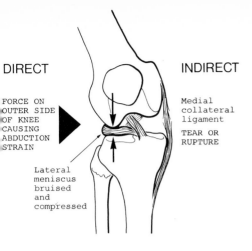

DIRECT

FORCE ON
OUTER SIDE
OF KNEE
CAUSING
ABDUCTION
STRAIN

Lateral
meniscus
bruised
and
compressed

INDIRECT

Medial
collateral
ligament

TEAR OR
RUPTURE

Figure 47. A blow on the outer side of the right knee, causing a direct injury to the outer side and an indirect injury to the inner side.

joint. This denotes a ligamentous rupture which requires operative treatment. However, the majority of these cases are moderate to severe and most authorities will treat them in a plaster cast from mid-thigh to mid-calf for periods varying from four to eight weeks with the knee in slight flexion. The patient should be instructed regarding carrying out isometric exercises in the plaster of Paris cast.

The following method has been found to be most rewarding. An injection of 5 ml of one per cent xylocaine with 1 ml of Depomedrone is given into the tender point usually at the upper attachment of the ligament, just below the adductor tubercle. An Elastoplast dressing with a thick compression pad is placed over the point of injection and a plaster of Paris cast is put on with the knee in as full extension as possible. If applied soon after the injury any associated muscle spasm is overcome by the injection or, if it is not completely overcome, a wax bath and ultrasound before the plaster of Paris is applied; also, spraying the tender area with ethyl chloride or a cooling aerospray helps to relax the muscles on the inner side of the knee. If extension of the injured knee is still not full, the heel should be put on a firm object so that when the leg is elevated the weight of the leg will gradually help to straighten the knee as its weight coaxes the muscles to relax.

As soon as the plaster has been applied and allowed to dry, isometric exercises are started and carried out at hourly intervals throughout the day. The following day the plaster is split down the front and the patient starts home treatment four times daily with twice daily physiotherapy out of the plaster. Often flexion of the knee is painful and difficult at first but with ice packs and the physiotherapy, including very gently rotary manipulative movements, progress is soon made, particularly when the tender ligamentous and tendonous structures pass over the tender bony medial condyle. It is often found when this happens that flexion suddenly improves appreciably, but in trying to establish extension again there is return of pain until the strapping muscles pass back over the tender point in the ligament. If treated gently as above there is usually sufficient flexion after five days to allow exercise on either a stationary or ordinary bicycle.

Unless operation is indicated, injury to the medial collateral ligament is always treated in this way, but two examples show the difference between starting treatment soon after injury compared with commencing on the twelfth day after injury.

EXAMPLE 1

A varsity player sustained a typical medial collateral injury to the left knee. He was examined on the third day after injury and treatment was started immediately as advised above. By the sixth day he was able to start using a bicycle and by the tenth day was able to train vigorously. As he was wanted for the Oxford and Cambridge match to be played on the seventeenth day after injury, he was asked to play for a London club side exactly fourteen days after the injury. He came through well and played in the varsity match without recurrence of his injury.

EXAMPLE 2

Another player had a similar injury to the right knee and was not seen until the twelfth day after injury, when the knee was flexed to 15°, that is to say, full extension lacked 15° and he had only about 20° of active flexion. After an injection and concentrated treatment he made slow progress for a week, but after a further injection on the nineteenth day, he made such rapid improvement that he was able to start training on the twenty-first day and played in a practice match on exactly the twenty-eighth day after injury, and a representative match exactly five weeks after the injury.

Treated in this way, the risk of bone forming in the ligament as in Pellegrini–Stieda ossification is completely eradicated. So often these cases are advised to rest in plaster of Paris for four to eight weeks and it is often a further several months before they are symptom-free. During the vigorous approach to the treatment of medial collateral injuries, the patient must steel himself to suffer a certain amount of pain in carrying out

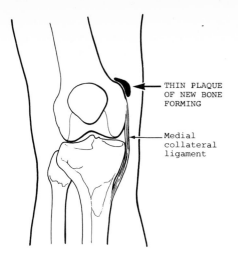

THIN PLAQUE
OF NEW BONE
FORMING

Medial
collateral
ligament

Figure 48. Pelegrini-Stieda ossification as a complication of a medial collateral ligament injury.

exercises of a non-straining nature. Although exercising in this way may cause some pain, provided the exercises are non weight-bearing, no harm is done.

2(b). Rupture of the Medial Collateral Ligament

Often the player is found lying on the ground with the lower leg below the knee at a marked outward angle to the femur. There may be little pain and no marked swelling. The deformity should be corrected and first-aid carried out with splints and bandages.

Operation is indicated as soon as circumstances permit perfect conditions. At operation it will be found that the medial compartment of the knee opens and the anterior cruciate ligament and medial meniscus can easily be examined. In some cases, where there is a frank lesion of the medial meniscus, it should be removed, and a tear or rupture of the anterior cruciate ligament repaired if feasible. The medial collateral ligament is carefully repaired and the knee held in plaster for three weeks in 10° of flexion. Isometric exercises are started the following day and should be carried out hourly for two minutes throughout the day. These include both flexion and extension exercises against the resistance of the plaster. After removal of the stitches in three weeks, the patient can be allowed to exercise out of the plaster, which has been split, carrying out only flexion and extension exercises. Physiotherapy should also be given daily and walking allowed in plaster with crutches. It will be noted that flexion returns to normal quickly provided isometric exercises have been performed conscientiously from the second day. Full movements and good

157

muscle control should be present after six weeks with walking with sticks or crutches out of plaster, but with Robert Jones bandage support. Return to full athletic activities should be possible within four months.

3. Meniscus Injuries

The meniscii are liable to injuries of a rotation nature associated with flexion or extension at the same time. The medial meniscus is stated to be liable to injury three to four times as frequently as the lateral meniscus, but this varies in different statistical reviews. Pathological conditions of the lateral meniscus are often silent though may give rise to conflicting symptoms. The symptoms may be caused by a congenital discoid lateral meniscus, or one in which cystic degeneration has occurred.

A history of the knee giving way and locking, a positive McMurray, 'click clonk and catch' on rotation, the position of tender points usually makes the diagnosis of a torn medial meniscus relatively easy. Recent advances in joint radiography and radioscopy have helped to clarify doubtful cases and should be employed in those cases in which the diagnosis is not clear or absolute. It is very disconcerting to remove a torn medial meniscus and to find later there was involvement of the lateral meniscus as well.

There are differences of opinion as to how much of the meniscus should be removed. Usually, if it is the first episode of locking and there is a straightforward vertical split of the meniscus with displacement medially into the joint, most surgeons are satisfied to remove only the displaced anterior portion of the meniscus. This procedure affects the joint minimally and recovery is rapid. Often the player may return to competitive sport in six to eight weeks.

On the other hand, if there have been several episodes of locking over a period of over three months and on operation the meniscus is found not only split but also contused and ragged, partly posteriorly, it is best to remove the whole meniscus.

An extended period of convalescence is essential to allow good healing to occur in this type of case, especially if there has been an associated osteochondritis of any severity. Although quadriceps exercises are started the day after operation, weight-bearing on the joint is not allowed for at least three weeks and then carefully graduated. It may be three to four months before the player can return to competitive sport; much longer if there has been an associated chondromalacia patellae or osteochondritis.

4. Enlargement of the Fatty Pads

This is common in females with a tendency to genu recurvatum and chondromalacia patellae. It is often part of a swollen knee as the result of a direct blow on the patella and surrounding tissues as occurs after a fall. They are often made symptom-free by conservative methods though sometimes operative removal of the fatty pads is necessary.

Conservative treatment should be tried first and should consist of raising both heels to 4 cm (Cuban type), short-wave, friction massage, ultrasound and injections of xylocaine one per cent 2 mls, hydrocortisone 1 ml at weekly intervals, four applications if necessary. If symptoms persist for more than two months, operative removal of large portions of the fatty pads is indicated.

5. Chondromalacia Patellae and Osteochondritis of the Femoral Condyles

These conditions may occur together or separately. An area of cartilage erosion on the articular surface of the patella may correspond with one on the femoral medial condyle. There may be a definite history of an accident in which the patella attempted to sublux or dislocate and an osteochondral fracture has occurred.

In fact it would seem there are two definite varieties of the two conditions: the first, in which subluxation or dislocation of the patella does not take place, has often been found to be associated with tightness of the corresponding hip muscles with limitation of hip movements and genu valgum; the second in which subluxation and dislocation of the patella does occur but also has the same tightness of hip movements, genu valgum and a laterally placed tibial tuberosity as well.

The first type often improves with concentrated physiotherapy, compensation for the genu valgum with an inner wedge to the heel and tread of the shoes combined with exercises and manipulations to restore full hip movements. These conservative procedures should be given a good trial before operation is considered, unless on radiography there is present a large area of erosion or a loose piece of cartilage from an osteochondral fracture.

Sometimes a relatively simple procedure is advocated by Helal of splitting the lateral fibrous capsule, including the expansion of the vastus lateralis. This is sufficient, combined, if necessary, with smoothing down or eradicating any osteochondral roughness.

The release of the lateral quadriceps and capsule expansion as originally advocated by Emslie and recommended by Helfet, and the transfer of the tibial tuberosity and tightening or overlapping of the medial capsule, should be reserved for those cases in which subluxation and dislocation take place constantly. Transfer of the tibial tuberosity should never be carried out until after the upper tibial epiphysis has closed.

Cases in which there is marked osteochondral fibrillation (worn cartilage on the ends of the bones) may take months to heal and the sportsman may be forced to give up his sports at least for a year until the area has completely healed.

6. General Joint Laxity: the Unstable Knee

Severely damaged knees in which there has been a subluxation or dislocation of the knee itself, with severe stretching or rupture of the corresponding ligament, present a difficult problem in restoring the stability of the knee so that the sportsman can return to strenuous exercise.

It may be obvious that operative reconstruction of ligaments is necessary. Sometimes a well-fitting knee brace, so that graduated exercises can be combined with vigorous home treatment and physiotherapy, is helpful. Helfet has produced a superb knee support which can be worn during strenuous games. Of course internal derangements, loose bodies, subluxing patellae must be carefully excluded; all of these can give rise to an unstable knee in which there is locking, catching or momentary giving way of the knee.

There are groups of cases which follow injuries of moderate to severe degree in which the quadriceps and surrounding muscles have been allowed to waste and lose their proper extensibility and contractibility. Adhesions may have formed and require even manipulation under anaesthesia to break them down. These procedures must be followed by further graduated exercises and physiotherapy including progressive manipulations until full movements and muscle power are restored. More commonly, however, this type of case follows meniscectomy of either the medial or both. A typical example is given.

EXAMPLE

In an international rugby football player both meniscii had been removed from the right knee in 1971, the first in May and the second in October. Following these procedures the knee tended to swell and movement was limited. It was just impossible for him to return to rugby football as every

160

time he practised the knee became painful and swollen. There was a considerable amount of synovial thickening and swelling with limitation of extremes of movement, particularly flexion. There was slightly increased movement in both antero-posterior and lateral directions: this is commonly seen after removal of both meniscii.

The patient was given instructions as to carrying out home treatment and advised to do this conscientiously. One month later a manipulation under anaesthetic was performed and at the same time 10 mls of one per cent xylocaine and 1 ml of Depomedrone were injected into the knee joint. A further injection was given two weeks later.

The patient made such a marked improvement that he has been able to play first-class rugby for the last three seasons. In his case exercises were graduated carefully, he did his other 'homework' religiously and had physiotherapy daily. Slocombe repair operation is a useful procedure in those in which there is a laxity of medial collateral ligament with increased lateral rotation of the tibia. At operation a sheet of the fascial attachment of the sartorius is turned up and over from above and posterior to its insertion into the tibia, and sutured to the medial femoral joint capsule. This has the effect of tightening up the medial side of the knee.

7. Lateral Pivot Shift

This occurs often enough to be recorded as an interesting phenomenon. It has been described by MacIntosh of Toronto following injuries to the knee sufficiently severe to cause stretching or rupture of the anterior cruciate ligament and tears of the medial meniscus particularly.

At 30° flexion of the knee with the weight load on the lateral compartment of the knee – as occurs when the foot becomes firmly planted to make a sudden turn or stop – there is a forward subluxation of the lateral femoral condyle. A snap reduction takes place when the knee gives in further flexion. The patient feels as if the knee goes out or comes apart. This snap is due to the ilio-tibial band jumping forwards or backwards over the lateral femoral condyle and can be dramatically cured by reefing the ilio-tibial band.

A strip of the ilio-tibial is dissected upwards and its base is left attached below. This strip is threaded round the front of the band, brought around the lateral collateral ligament and looped around it and then sutured to its bed. This has the effect of holding the lateral collateral ligament and band forwards thus preventing the forward subluxation of the lateral tibial condyle. In some cases lesions of lateral meniscus give symptoms similar to this derangement and removal of the meniscus is probably sufficient. However, this type of case may also be associated with osteochondral (ends of bones) erosion and this complication often means that the sportsman may be prevented from continuing, at least for many months, until the eroded articular surface has healed.

8. Derangement of the Medial Tibio-femoral Compartment in the Older Sportsman

This occurs in the older athlete when early osteoarthritis is setting in. The medial compartment of the joint often gives rise to a tender, slightly swollen, painful knee over the front and inner side. These cases are aggravated by playing golf or shooting over rough ground. Many of them get better gradually with modified rest, twice-daily home treatment, and four to six injections, with physiotherapy three times a week.

In certain cases, before advising operation, a manipulation of the knee under anaesthetic sometimes helps the condition by breaking down adhesions. Vigorous after-treatment should follow until there is full painless movement. This is the type of knee condition which, if a conservative approach is continued, eventually becomes symptom-free.

Before subjecting the patient to an operation, both an arthrograph and an arthroscopy should be considered. Helfet considers these cases should be subjected to operation early, as he considers the lesion of the meniscus contributes to increasing irreversible damage to the joint. Some cases are associated with transverse splits of the medial meniscus and even contusion and fraying of the whole meniscus, particularly posteriorly. These pathological conditions will be picked up and removal of the meniscus becomes a necessity, because it causes constant internal derangement of the joint.

Goodbody, on the other hand, is in favour of caution in the removal of the meniscus, as it acts as a buffer between the ends of the femur and tibia. The need for operation is then only considered necessary in those cases in which continual derangement of the knee occurs with locking.

The Thigh, Hip Joint and Pelvis

Contusions and tears of the thigh muscles can lead to disabilities which can

162

keep the sportsmen away from sport for months unless properly treated.

Haematoma formation deep in the front of the thigh in relation to the quadriceps can lead to myositis ossificans (Figure 50).

Recurrent tears of the rectus femoris are extremely difficult as they seem to be associated with 'tight hips'. Many sportsmen are born with 'tight hips' and this condition may be present on one side only. Even young athletes have been examined who are constantly sustaining injuries on one side in the form of strains, tears and bursitis in the groin and around the greater trochanter, and it has been found on examination that they have a 'tight hip' only on the side prone to injury. In many cases there is a swelling in the middle of the front of the thigh where the rectus femoris merges with the vastus intermedius (middle of thigh). It would seem that recurrences keep on taking place until there is complete separation of the rectus from the vastus intermedius, forming a definite break in the musculature of the thigh, and sometimes a hole in the middle of the thigh. If a sportsman is treated by the AT Approach method, and if he still has symptoms at the end of a month, the thigh muscles must be stretched thoroughly under an anaesthetic, to obtain as full movement as possible in the knee and hip joints. Injections of xylocaine and urea and salicyclic acid are given at the same time.

Figure 49. How a haematoma will gravitate and cause a synovial effusion.

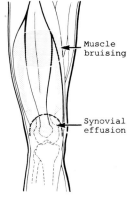

Muscle bruising

Synovial effusion

THE HAMSTRINGS

Tears of the hamstrings can be mild, moderate or severe. Moderate to severe tears are notorious for giving rise to recurrences. This often is because strenuous exercise is undertaken before the torn muscle has recovered its length and strength. As in the case of tears of the quadriceps, tears of the hamstrings seem to occur in sportsmen with 'tight hips'. It would seem obvious if the muscles are short and contracted, as they are in 'tight hips', that when they are overstretched they are more likely to strain or tear. If the tear is moderate to severe a reactionary mass of torn muscle fibres, haematoma and exudate will form at the point of tear, which may, in the case of semitendinosus and semimembranosus, occur anywhere along their course at the top, middle or lower end. In the case of the biceps femoris the short head often tears, and, if put to strain too soon, the long head suffers injury later.

These cases are examples where good treatment – Ice, Compression and Elevation – should be started as soon as possible, followed by graduated exercise, ultrasound and faradic stimulation to all the hamstrings. If bruising after a few days appears down the calf and around the ankle, this is a good sign.

These cases are often seen several days after injury in which no treatment has been given, and then an injection of 10 ml one per cent xylocaine and 10 ml of urea and salicyclic acid is indicated with a view to breaking up the mass of blood clot and disorientated muscle fibres. This injection is followed immediately by physiotherapy twice daily. In all cases, weight-bearing exercises may have to be modified according to progress, and sticks and crutches may be necessary. The patient himself should carry out home treatment at least twice daily. By the end of three weeks full extensibility of the muscle should have been obtained and training started. If one month after injury there is still restriction of movement, careful manipulative stretching of the muscle under a general anaesthetic should be carried out, followed by further physiotherapy and graduated exer-

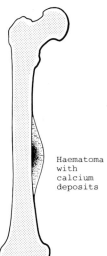

Figure 50. How deep bruising in the muscles associated with the femur can cause periosteal stripping and an organising haematoma resulting in myositis ossificans.

Haematoma
with
calcium
deposits

cises. The sportsman with tears of any severity may not be able to take part in vigorous competitive sport for six weeks, and two months in those who have undergone a manipulation under anaesthesia. During this time gentle manipulative stretching of all the hip structures should be carried out so as to overcome the restriction of a 'tight hip' joint, and restore full length and strength to the torn muscle. So often, however, contraction and shortening of these muscles are part of a 'tight hip' complaint, and unless the joint movements are increased to normal there will be constant recurrence.

THE PELVIS

The pelvis consists of the sacrum at the back and the innominate bones on each side meeting in front at the junction of both pubic rami, in the symphysis pubis. The innominate bone on each side is made up of the ilium, ischium and pubic bones.

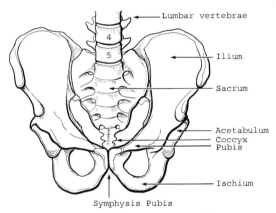

Figure 51. Front view of pelvis.

THE HIP JOINT

The hip joint is a typical ball-and-socket joint, and has a large articular surface. The head of the femur articulates with the acetabulum, which consists of contributions from the ilium, ischium and pubis.

The capsule of the hip joint is strengthened by three strong ligaments: the anterior (iliofemoral or ligament of Bigelow); the posterior ischiofemoral; and the medial pubofemoral.

The range of hip movements, because it is a ball-and-socket joint, is

165

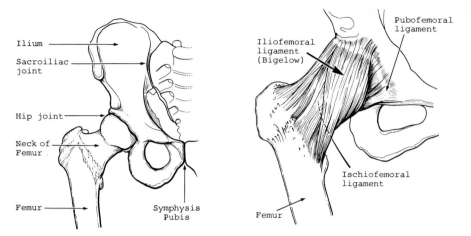

Left: Figure 52. Front view of right hip with right side of pelvis.
Right: Figure 53. Front view of right hip with ligaments.

global or in every direction. From the neutral position with the leg straight 0° to full flexion is 120°. Extension is from 0° to 30° or less. Rotation in flexion at 90°. Inward (internal) is 35° average and outward (external) is 35° average. Adduction is from 0–35°. Abduction is from 0–45°.

As in most cases the acetabular fossa surrounds a large portion of the femoral head, this makes subluxations and dislocations difficult. Subluxations and dislocations that do occur are usually the result of violent injury and are often associated with fractures of the acetabulum. If these are present with displacement of fragments, accurate operative reconstruction of the acetabular fossa is essential, otherwise osteoarthritis will appear early in life.

After reduction, whether fractures are present or not, strong traction must be applied as continuously as possible for at least one month. While in traction, exercises are carried out several times daily, and physiotherapy should also be given daily with ultrasound, massage and faradism. The traction may be allowed off for toilet purposes in certain cases without fracture. At the end of a month hot baths and free exercises on the bed are allowed, and intermittent skin traction is carried out daily. This can be done by leaving the cover to the sticky surface of the Elastoplast extension and bandaging it on firmly so that it can be removed easily and used

166

dozens of times. At the end of six weeks partial weight-bearing with crutches is started, but full weight-bearing is not allowed for four months. Osteoarthritis of the injured hip joint is liable at a later date, but an active regime of home treatment will help to check its appearance, and may arrest and postpone it indefinitely if the patient is conscientious in a daily progressive regime of exercises.

THE SACROILIAC JOINT

The sacroiliac joint consists of three parts: an oblique upper portion which articulates with the upper articular surface of the ilium and in which there is a synovial cavity: an intermediate part with no synovial cavity; and a lower vertical portion also lined with synovial membrane.

Sacroiliac strain or subluxation used frequently to be the diagnosis of low back pain before 1934. In most cases the correct diagnosis now is a facet joint syndrome at the L.5/S.1 facet joint on the painful side. For the diagnosis to be made some of the following sacroiliac tests must be positive:
1. Mennell's Test.
   (a) Pain on forcing the anterior superior iliac spines outwards. This puts pressure and strain on the anterior sacroiliac capsule.
   (b) Pain on compressing the anterior superior iliac spines forward and inwards. Pressure is applied to the posterior sacroiliac ligaments and they show symptoms and signs of injury.
2. In the lateral lying position pain must be experienced over the sacro-iliac joints on abduction of the upper leg.
3. Baer's Tender Point which is just inside McBurney's Point and denotes tenderness of the anterior capsule.

Last stated that the sacroiliac strain was uncommon and only occurred in relation to pregnancy in women when the sacroiliac ligaments were lax, and in both sexes only when the patient has landed on the feet from great heights. Often a sacroiliac subluxation is diagnosed without positive tests. Muscle spasm from L.5/S.1 facet joint involvement will often make the pelvis tilt on one side and the bones of the sacroiliac joint become prominent on that side. Mistakes are sometimes made because the insertion of the muscles is over the posterior surface of the sacroiliac and ligaments which are in relation to the joint become tender.

In true sacroiliac strain, examination of the joint by digital pressure

167

through the rectum reveals tenderness of the anterior capsule when the ilium has been forced backwards.

Treatment by short-wave, ultrasound using a special adaptor, massage through the rectum, with manipulations, will be successful in most cases. When the posterior capsule is involved the ilium having been forced forwards, the same type of physiotherapy combined with injections usually improves the condition.

SYMPHYSIS PUBIS

Inflammatory changes in the cartilage of the symphysis pubis have recently been reported in sufficient numbers of cases for the profession to study them in detail. Factors maybe contributing to this condition have been found to include:

(a) Strains of pyramidalis and rectus abdominus at their insertions into the symphysis pubis. Fast bowlers and footballers suffer these, and in many cases it is found that when they are flexing their spinal column forward they are not checking and resisting the movement by synergic contraction of the abdominal muscles. In the action of a fast bowling the abdominal muscles should act as a break to the forward movement of the trunk. The forward movement of the spine and the pelvis should be in as straight a line as possible. The movement is then through the hip joint, otherwise the anterior abdominal muscles are slack and strains take place at the symphysis pubis.

(b) In several cases it has been found that the patient with a painful symphysis pubis has been suffering from a urethritis in which B. Coli (bacteria from the colon) has been isolated. Most cases clear up with attention to postural training and elimination of the urethritis if present.

Bone grafting of the symphysis pubis which is advocated by some orthopaedic surgeons does not seem to be logical. Cases of complete disruption of the symphysis pubis associated with fractures of the pelvis have been seen, in which the patients have been able to execute double somersaults after six months. If they are able to accomplish this feat it would seem that to immobilise the symphysis completely is not necessary to cure the chondritis (inflammation of the cartilage).

However, rest over a long period of about six months has resulted in a cure and therefore results claimed by the insertion of a bone block may be attributed to the prolonged post-operative rest.

168

Back and Neck, Concussion and Rib Cage Injuries

It is necessary to have a clear grasp of the separate parts which combine to make up the components of each spinal segment and to understand that injuries to these structures depend on the initial severity of the injury, age of the sportsman, his general posture and whether he executes his actions correctly. The presence of a gouty diathesis or toxic focus must also be borne in mind, particularly if the condition does not respond to treatment quickly.

Altogether, there are thirty-four vertebrae, but only twenty-two discs, the first being between C.2 and 3 and the last between L.5 and S.1. The various entities of a spinal segment with its spinal nerve roots on each side consist of:

(a) the vertebral body;

(b) the intervertebral disc between the anterior and posterior longitudinal ligaments which join adjacent vertebral bodies together;

(c) cartilaginous rings placed on the upper and lower border of each vertebral body. Each disc is separated from the vertebral body above and below by a cartilaginous ring and it is through it that the nucleus pulposus derives its blood supply. Therefore the joint between adjacent vertebral bodies is of a cartilaginous type and allows little movement, but it is the sum total of these which accounts for the full range of spinal movements. Each disc consists of two parts: the annulus fibrosus; the nucleus pulposus. Excluding the first two vertebrae, the intervertebral discs comprise about one quarter of the length of the spinal column. The annulus fibrosus is intimately connected with the cartilaginous plates of the vertebral bodies above and below and the anterior and posterior longitudinal ligaments in front and behind. It consists of laminated fibrous tissue and fibro-cartilage, and surrounds the nucleus pulposus situated half way between the posterior longitudinal ligament and the centre of the annulus fibrosus. The nucleus pulposus consists of a soft, pulpy, highly elastic substance of yellowish colour and has a direct connection with the blood supply of the vertebral body;

(d) the transverse process;

(e) the pedicles;

(f) the intervertebral or facet joints, superior and inferior, with cap-

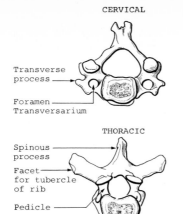

CERVICAL

Transverse process

Foramen Transversarium

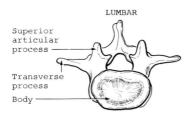

THORACIC

Spinous process

Facet for tubercle of rib

Pedicle

LUMBAR

Superior articular process

Transverse process

Body

Figure 54. Typical cervical, thoracic and lumbar vertebrae. The facet, intervertebral or apophyseal upper articulations differ. The cervical are flat and transverse, the thoracic are oblique, while the lumbar are vertical.

sular synovia and ligaments between the adjacent vertebrae;

(g) the laminae joining to form (h);

(h) the spinous processes.

In the dorsal region each vertebra has two articular facets, one on the side of the body and one on the transverse process for the ribs (see Figure 55).

In each vertebra the pedicles and laminae form the neural arches. Overlying the spinal segment are the corresponding spinal muscles which function in the act of fixing and moving the spinal column. Injury or disease can attack any of these entities of a spinal segment, either separately or together.

If the injury is relatively slight, the muscles may have been stretched, or at worst a few fibres may have been torn. A more severe type of injury will strain, stretch or tear the muscle, and if not completely absorbed by the muscular layers will pass on to the deeper joint structures with involvement of the ligaments, disc and even bony elements, particularly the facet or intervertebral joints. In the lumbar region the patient may therefore suffer from so-called 'lumbago', due to protective spasm of the lumbar muscles, and even a type of secondary sciatica due to the involvement of the segmental nerve.

There are three levels where more mobile sections of the spine join the more stable ones. Firstly, at the top of the spinal column where the occiput (base of the skull) moves on the atlas (the first vertebra); the atlanto-occipital joint (the first spinal joint) plays an important part in flexion and extension of the head. Rotation of the head on the neck occurs mainly between the atlas and axis (second spinal vertebra) and, to a lesser extent, in the lower cervical joints. The second level is at the lower cervical area, at C.5 and C.6., and involving C.6 and C.7 and C.7 and D.1 where the cervico-scapular muscles are attached to the upper extremity of the spine. The third level is in the lumbar region, L.4, L.5, S.1., where the trunk is attached to the pelvis.

The spinal nerves can become involved by stretching or fibrosis taking place at the muscle origins from the vertebrae or more commonly by root cuff fibrosis. This signifies fibrous changes from trauma occurring in the pia arachnoid sheath (tissue covering the spinal cord) at the beginning of each spinal nerve as it travels from the spinal cord out through its corresponding spinal foramina. At all levels the facet or posterior intervertebral joints are likely to be involved. In the cervical spine there are the joints of Lushka at the back of each vertebral body, which can undergo osteoarthritic changes following injury. Poor posture and the incorrect execution of movements in everyday life can also in time produce gradual degenerative changes. These changes can irritate the spinal cord as well as the nerve roots and cause cervical torticollis (muscle spasm) with pain, headaches and restriction of movements, and possibly pain in the shoulder girdle and down the arm.

Throughout the dorsal spine there is limited movement of the spinal vertebrae. There are extra costo-vertebral and costo-transverse joints on both sides and injury to these can be associated with fibrositic changes in the corresponding overlying muscles, ligaments and along the nerves.

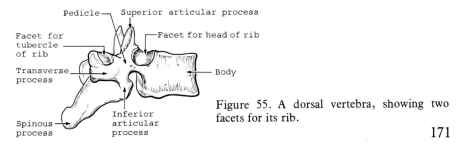

Figure 55. A dorsal vertebra, showing two facets for its rib.

171

Pain, particularly on exercise, is often quite severe due to involvement of these joints and their spinal nerves. There may be pain radiating around the rib cage to the front of the chest and abdomen as well.

Involvement of the facet or intervertebral joints of the lumbar spine will also cause protective muscle spasm.

Injury, especially if combined with degenerative changes in the disc and spinal joints, can cause the following entities:

1. Muscular strains and tears of the cervical, dorsal and lumbar muscles. Treatment is the same as in muscular injuries in other parts of the body.

2. Strains and sprains of the facet or intervertebral joints.

3. Disc involvement resulting in first swelling of nucleus pulposus then bulging in front of the posterior longitudinal ligament and finally rupture of the posterior longitudinal ligament with fragmented pieces of the disc substance going into the spinal canal and probably pressing on nerve roots, giving rise to a true sciatica (pain down the leg to the foot).

4. Spondylosis and spondylolisthesis.

At all stages the AT Approach to treatment should be instigated and should consist of the following:

1. The right amount of rest according to the severity of the condition and the symptoms.

2. Support: collars for cervical spine with universal slings if necessary to support the arm and thus prevent strain on the cervical muscles and joints; rib cage splints for dorsal spine; corsets, plaster of Paris casts, a Gauvain brace or McKee brace for dorso-lumbar and lumbar spine. The corsets may be re-inforced by firm bandaging with elastic webbing.

3. Injections of xylocaine, urea and salicyclic solution, Depomedrone locally.

4. Physiotherapy – short-wave, ultrasound, interferential, massage and gentle progressive manipulations, combined with traction if indicated. In cases not recovering quickly, manipulation under an anaesthetic should be considered combined with an epidural injection.

If poor posture and badly executed movements are present, they combine to worsen the injury process and naturally the reaction to it is more liable to be of greater severity. In many cases without injury the result of poor posture and habitually bad execution of movements, has produced an underlying condition of a fibrositic nature which, though not sufficient in itself to produce symptoms, lies dormant until a definite injury sets in motion a severe reaction out of all proportion to the degree of the injury. The late Hume Kendall taught that back exercises should be considered under the initials LIFE (Lumbar; Isometric; Flexion; Exercise).

T'ai Chi Ch'uan, the ancient Chinese method of exercises including back bending, was always done with a straight back so that the trunk and pelvis were held rigid and flexion took place through the hip joint. There is a great revival of these exercises today. Active Alerted Posture, good back posture, simulates these ancient methods exactly. Flexion of the spine is never allowed to take place at the lumbo-sacral level, but through the hip joints, so that this vulnerable level is never subjected to strain and the chance of disc involvement is lessened.

In these cases the AT Approach should be started immediately. If the reaction is severe, rest and support or even complete bed rest may be necessary. Hot and cold rough towel compresses four times daily for fifteen minutes will help absorb the inflammatory reaction, combined with massage of sufficient depth and type as required, as well as two of the following: ultrasound, short-wave, interferential, faradism and very gentle manipulations. These usually help to relax the muscle spasms.

Some authorities consider that there is inevitable disc involvement where there is pronounced muscle spasm, but in many cases the facet or intervertebral joints are the structures more often affected. If, however, severe muscle spasm is associated with sciatica, limited straight leg raising, lost or impaired reflexes and sensory changes, one of the discs is probably involved. Injections of 10 ml xylocaine one per cent and 10 ml of urea and salicylic acid with 2 ml of Depomedrone are inserted into the facet joint involved.

Athletes over forty-five who play tennis, golf and other relatively light sports may develop a type of sciatica of segmental distribution. This often signifies spondylosis, which means the corresponding disc may show degeneration but there are early osteoarthritic changes in the facet joints.

In the spine generally, if the combination of rest and the AT Approach, including gentle manipulation, do not succeed after a month, a controlled manipulation under general anaesthesia may be tried. In the lumbar region this may be performed in combination with an epidural injection and injection of the corresponding facet or intervertebral joints. Operative treatment is only considered after conservative treatment has been given a good trial, unless there is evidence of spinal nerve paralysis. If this state does not improve quickly or if a myelogram demonstrates the presence of a prolapsed disc, immediate operative removal of the offending disc is indicated. Some authorities consider that spinal fusion should be performed at the same time as the removal of the disc. However, this fusion should be considered only if the spinal segment appears unstable or if the patient is a manual labourer or his sport is of a violent nature such as football, weight-lifting or motor racing.

SPONDYLOSIS AND SPONDYLOLISTHESIS (LOW BACK PAIN)

These conditions occur in sportsmen sufficiently often to be included.

Newman's classic paper (1963) describes five different grades.

Grade 1 is congenital and is a marked forward slip of lumbar 5 on sacral 1.

Grade 2 is the commonest one in sportsmen and although there may be a congenital weakness present it is considered by Newman and others to be due to stress or fatigue fracture in the pars interarticularis (in the low back). A cricket professional – fast bowler – showed no evidence of stress fracture on X-rays in July, whereas by October one was revealed in the pars interarticularis on one side only. After two months, further X-rays showed the condition present on the other side as well. After three months in plaster with isometric exercises, X-rays showed that the fractures were healing satisfactorily.

Grade 3 is rare and due to injury causing a fracture in the pars interarticularis and the pedicle.

Grade 4 is associated with osteoarthritis and degenerative changes in the older sportsman.

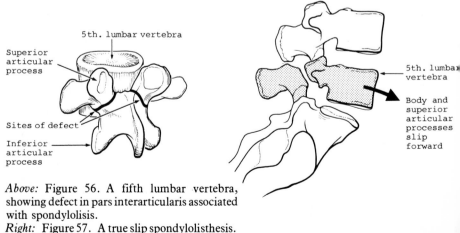

Above: Figure 56. A fifth lumbar vertebra, showing defect in pars interarticularis associated with spondylolisis.
Right: Figure 57. A true slip spondylolisthesis.

Grade 5 is due to a structural defect in the bone and is rare.

The important one for the sportsman is Grade 2. Some cases give rise to disabling symptoms and are a problem even in adolescence. When the symptoms commence and are severe enough to cause lack of function Buck recommends screw fixation of the fractured pars interarticularis sometimes combined with bone grafting.

A few cases giving rise to pain and sciatica with tenderness of the tissues over the fracture site are made symptom-free by removing the loose laminae and the pars interarticularis up to the fracture. Pridie considered that the tissues of the false joint at the site of fracture produced granulation tissue which irritated the sciatic root.

In those with prolonged symptoms exclusion of a prolapsed disc must be made by myelography and if present must be removed and the involved segment fused to the vertebrae above and below by either the anterior or posteriolateral approach. However, some cases respond to conservative treatment of support in plaster for three months during which time all the muscles of the low back, buttock and abdomen are exercised isometrically against the resistance of the plaster.

Throughout, the benefits from Active Alerted Posture are stressed and it may be that if sportsmen who are subject to back stress particularly, were aware of the benefits of this posture and practised it fewer cases of the condition would require treatment.

FRACTURES INVOLVING THE VERTEBRAL COLUMN

The significance of these varies according to which segment or segments of the vertebral column are involved and if the spinal cord itself is damaged. Fractures or fracture/dislocations of the cervical spine and odontoid process may be fatal, especially if the spinal fracture is above the fifth cervical vertebra because the respiratory muscles can be involved. If dislocations are present and the patient survives, reduction by head traction must be carried out gradually and cautiously, followed by stabilisation in a Minerva plaster collar at first and spinal fusion later, if necessary.

However, fractures of the odontoid process of the axis (C.2) often remain unstable fractures after traction and they should be stabilised by grafting to atlas (C.1) and sometimes the occiput. Often, if the patient survives without paralysis, unstable fractures of the cervical spine require

175

grafting, and following successful operation a decision has to be made as to whether the athlete should return to his sport. In many cases the athlete considers 'once lucky, twice shy' and is content to give up violent sports.

Fracture and fracture/dislocation below the fifth cervical level may give rise to transverse spinal cord paralysis, the significance of which will depend on the spinal level involved. Survival to these injuries have been greatly enhanced by the modern methods of rehabilitation practised at Spinal Centres such as that at Stoke Mandeville.

Operations on spinal fractures between the fifth dorsal vertebra and the second lumbar vertebra have to be carried out with great caution because the circulation of this part of the spinal cord is so precarious. Spinal fusion can often be carried out posteriorly or by the more modern anterior approach without involving the spinal canal. Compression fractures of the upper dorsal vertebrae may be almost without symptoms because of the splinting effect of the rib cage, and are often only discovered after radiology. Those in the lower dorsal and upper lumbar spine, where there is more movement in the spinal segments, may have to be immobilised for a much longer period. Provided there is no spinal cord involvement, rest in bed with exercises in the supine position with physiotherapy for a month can make it possible to become ambulatory with the help of a split spinal plaster jacket on one side or a Gauvain brace. Either of these can be taken off for baths, exercises and physiotherapy. Return to sport varies in each case and sometimes whether the individual is a professional. Obviously no undue risk should be taken. However, if the sport in question is riding and if the AT Approach makes the rider completely symptom-free in six weeks, he may be able to race or ride with the aid of a support belt and reinforced with webbing.

FRACTURE OF THE TRANSVERSE PROCESS

The nature and length of disability will depend on whether there has been a hairline crack or small separation of the fracture in comparison with a complete separation of the outer end of the transverse process from its inner end. The first type is usually due to a moderate injury and causes a relatively small amount of reaction, whereas the second type with gross separation denotes a severe injury, not only to the transverse process but to the surrounding muscles. Complete rest in bed is usually indicated for three weeks, with support from a plaster cast or firm corset. The cast can

176

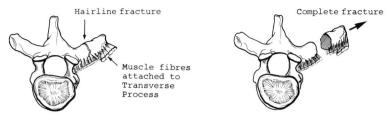

Figure 58. How a hairline fracture (above) differs from one with displacement. The former usually is symptom-free in two weeks, the latter in six weeks. Both these times depend on the case being treated by the Active Therapeutic Approach.

be split on one side after a few days to allow daily physiotherapy, and contrast baths and hot and cold towels may be applied to the injured area daily for twenty minutes. After treatment the split plaster is replaced and maintained in position with straps and elastic webbing. Isometric exercises against the resistance of the plaster cast are instigated from the beginning. Usually under this regime the patient is relatively symptom-free after three weeks and can return to full sporting activities with suitable support in eight weeks.

Jump jockeys have been treated who were found to have fractured their spine in a fall and continued to ride until forced to report – up to a week later. In such cases radiograph often reveals fractures involving sometimes two or three vertebrae. It is often the damage to the soft tissues causing tenderness and pain on movement which force the jockey to stop his activities and seek advice. A case of this type usually requires three week's complete rest in bed, sometimes in a plaster cast, which can be split and removed for contrast baths and physiotherapy. If there are no complications such as nerve root involvement or spinal instability, a corset can be substituted for the plaster cast after nine weeks and the jockey can return to jumping within three months. This will only happen if the soft tissue involvement is treated as seriously as the fractures by the AT Approach. Often a case of this type which has not had treatment for the soft tissue is seen six months after injury. Immediate treatment to both will hasten recovery in a relatively short time.

CONCUSSION
This is very common in boxing, steeplechasing, hunting, football and any sport where a fall on the head or a blow on the jaw will transmit impulses to

the base of the brain and cause contusion and bruising. Bleeding from nose, throat and ears must be noted. The patient should be under careful supervision for the next forty-eight hours at least. If there is a period of unconsciousness, he should be watched continuously during it and afterwards, and frequent checks must be made of the rate of breathing, pulse rate, size of pupil (whether equal and reacting to light) and reflexes generally and whether the state of the muscle tone is normal. If any of these observations are irregular they must be reported immediately.

An intracranial haemorrhage affecting the posterior meningeal artery can be silent for a long period, but suddenly give signs and symptoms which unless heeded at once can lead to a fatality. In a case such as this the patient should be situated near to a theatre with this kind of emergency in mind as it is essential to work quickly to stop the bleeding in the posterior meningeal artery, otherwise the intracranial pressure increases quickly with resultant death of the sportsman. If the loss of consciousness has been more than just momentary it is wise to advise complete rest for three weeks.

A rugby footballer experienced a period of unconsciousness for two and a half hours following a fall on the chin. Luckily, if there was any intracranial bleeding, it stopped. However, he took no care afterwards with the result that six months later he suffered from intractable headaches and a herpetic rash on the course of the facial nerve, which even to the present day tends to appear in cold weather.

Every sportsman, if concussed, should be treated in the following way: the approach to this condition in boxing should be copied. If consciousness is lost, a boxer is not allowed to return to his sport for at least one month, and if a second instance occurs an electro-encephalogram test must be normal before he is allowed to compete again. However, he must stop boxing for three months. After a third instance he is laid off for a whole year and must undergo an intensive examination before he is allowed to box again.

INJURIES TO THE THORACIC WALL AND RIB CAGE, INCLUDING FRACTURES

Contusion and bruising of the soft tissues as well as tears or strains of the muscles from the rib can be as painful as fractures of the ribs themselves. If severe or associated with fractures, the patient suffers great pain,

178

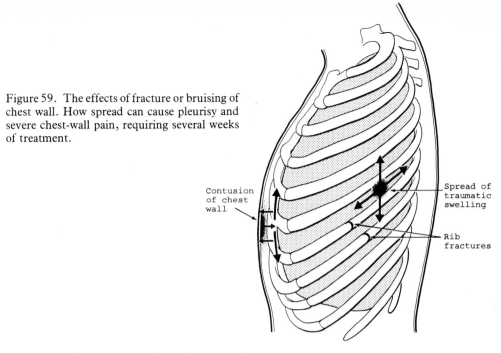

Figure 59. The effects of fracture or bruising of chest wall. How spread can cause pleurisy and severe chest-wall pain, requiring several weeks of treatment.

Contusion of chest wall

Spread of traumatic swelling

Rib fractures

especially if he tries to sit up from the lying position. A monkey pole to help him pull himself up with his arms is essential. If the muscles are torn or there are a limited number of fractures of the ribs, two or three injection of 10–20 mls of xylocaine into the painful areas daily can be of great benefit.

Support is controversial; some physicians consider it restricts the lung expansion on the good side. However, from personal experience, having sustained fractures of several ribs, severe contusions of the chest wall and even a split fracture of the sternum throughout its whole length – some of these on three separate occasions – there is no question that rib cage support makes all the difference to the comfort of the patient and at the same time allows him to breathe against its resistance and in fact allows greater expansion of the injured side. Strapping support is cumbersome and painful to remove and the best is a rib cage elastic support held with Velcro. It can be reinforced by several yards of elastic webbing placed over it. Both can be easily removed for baths and physiotherapy. Deep breathing exercises in a full bath of hot water is indicated and relatively easy to perform as the negative pressure inside the pleural cavity is balanced by the positive pressure outside.

179

It will be observed in bruising and contusion of the ribs that the products of haematoma seep and spread along the rib cage in all directions forwards, backwards, inwards and outwards. The inward spread may irritate the pleural surface and cause a traumatic pleurisy.

The AT Approach is essential and with suitable exercises, massage and ultrasound, in a few days the change in the amount of pain and other symptoms will be enormous. Unless this approach is adopted, symptoms of pain on deep breathing with tenderness of the tissues around the site of injury will probably persist for six to eight weeks, particularly if associated with fractures of the ribs.

The Upper Extremity

THE FINGERS, HAND, WRIST AND FOREARM

The joints of the wrist, hand and fingers are almost as numerous as those in the ankle and foot. Altogether there are twenty-nine joints of various varieties.

Direct Injuries

Contusions and bruises of these joints are frequent, due to direct injuries caused in boxing, by falls, strikes, balls or sticks, or by contact with other players. They must be treated urgently with contact baths, exercises, wax baths and, particularly, ultrasound. Contusion and bruising of the small joints, phalanges, metacarpo-phalangeal and carpo-metacarpal joints often require prolonged treatment, which can be prevented if the AT Approach is commenced immediately after the accident. Sometimes repeated injection of one per cent xylocaine 2 ml and Depomedrone 1 ml is necessary, combined with ultrasound, wax baths and friction massage. If the case has been allowed to become chronic, sometimes it takes six to eight weeks of concentrated treatment to be restored to normal, and will eventually respond only if the treatment has been given daily, combined with several injections at intervals.

If a fracture is present, and there is severe contusion and bruising as well, it is often best to treat the contusion and bruising first; and when there is full movement and restoration of normal conditions of the soft tissues then the fracture may be mobilised in a plaster cast, if necessary. In many cases the soft tissue injury will take less than a week of treatment before the plaster cast can be applied.

X-ray films must be taken in four planes. This is essential as fractures of the carpal scaphoid, dislocations of the semi-lunar and hairline fractures may be missed. In some cases, if a fracture is suspected but on the first X-ray there is no evidence of one, the films should be repeated in ten days' time when the fracture line may be more evident. In sports such as boxing it is extremely important in cases of fracture of the metacarpal shaft to restore perfect alignment, so that the knuckle line is normal, with no depression. If a deformity persists in the knuckle line, particularly in boxing, the function of the hand is definitely diminished. Reduction in these cases must be carried out either by traction and manipulation or by open operation. However, in many sports good function is obtained by simply protecting and supporting the fractured area for three weeks with a removable plaster cast or felt and bandages. At the same time, treatment of the overlying soft tissues twice daily is carried out, after removal of the protection and support.

Fractures of the shaft of the metatarsal bones, especially if transverse, must be considered to be serious, for although they may unite in time they may take several months to consolidate firmly. Re-fracture may occur if extra strain is placed on them too soon. Spiral fractures, however, usually unite quickly. If a transverse fracture in a boxer appears to be slow in uniting, freshening of the area of fracture with drilled holes and grafting with bone slivers may be indicated.

The treatment of fractured scaphoids is very controversial. Rigby-Jones, the orthopaedic surgeon, stated that he has never immobilised a fractured scaphoid in plaster. He had himself fractured both his scaphoids and treated them in a removable splint, taking them off to operate when necessary. Both joined perfectly by bony union, but in each case there had been no displacement of the fractured ends from the beginning.

In most cases the conventional method of treating fractured scaphoids with no displacement in a plaster cast is worth the eight to ten weeks it takes for union to be firm. The type of plaster cast is controversial. Some authorities believe that, provided the wrist is supported, union will occur whether the thumb is included in the plaster or not. On the Continent some authorities think that the plaster should include the elbow joint, as this will prevent pronation and supination, and therefore promote earlier

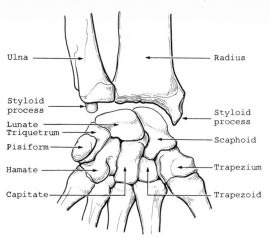

Figure 60. Front view of left wrist.

union. If plaster treatment is decided upon, the full cast above the elbow is best because it will ensure a quicker union. Isometric exercises are carried out in the cast. In the professional sportsman, however, consideration should be given as to the type of sport and work he requires to perform in the immediate future. Some fractures of the carpus associated with displacement of the scaphoid, transcarpal dislocation or both should be reduced immediately by open operation and grafting of the fracture, particularly if a small proximal fragment is present. Unless this is performed at once union will always be doubtful, and the fracture may take months to consolidate. With open operation and bone grafting, union should be complete in eight to ten weeks. However, if a professional steeplechase jockey fractures his scaphoid or a metacarpal bone in the middle of the season, his livelihood is threatened for at least three months. Fractures may then be treated as severe sprains of the hand and wrist, and a special wrist gauntlet worn whilst riding. However, in between racing he wears a split plaster cast. At the end of the racing season the fracture is reviewed and, if not united, grafting can be carried out then.

Dislocation of the semilunar bone occurs sufficiently frequently to warrant careful examination of X-rays in all cases of injury to the wrist. Reduction under full anaesthetic is possible in the early stages. The removal of the bone can give satisfactory results, but replacement by a silastic implant is more conventional today.

Late Cases of Non-Union of the Scaphoid

Excellent results have been obtained by removal of the scaphoid some twenty years after fracture. Some authorities replace this fractured scaphoid with a silastic implant and obtain excellent results. Unless the associated osteoarthritis of the wrist and other carpal joints, which is almost certain to be present, is made symptom-free before the operation, the results can be poor.

EXAMPLE

A prominent cricketer, captain of a minor county, fractured his left scaphoid at the age of eighteen. At thirty-eight he was beginning to experience pain and loss of wrist movement and strength. Osteoarthritic changes were present in the wrist and carpal joints. The scaphoid was removed, and early rehabilitation started. He claimed that for the subsequent six years after the operation he had batted better than ever before, with a higher average. Seen recently some twenty years after the operation the wrist and hand were functioning well.

Strains of the forearm and wrist tendons give rise to stenosing tenosynovitis, and these can be resistant to all forms of conservative treatment, and occasionally require surgical intervention. However, if the active therapeutic approach, including injections into the tendon sheath, is carried out, most cases recover relatively quickly.

Tenosynovitis of the tendons of the wrist can cause a period of prolonged disability. This applies particularly to the thumb extensors on the outer posterior aspect, and the extensor and flexor carpi ulnaris on the inner aspect. The latter occurs particularly in right-handed tennis players, and the left wrist in right-handed golfers. Injection therapy, wax baths, ultrasound and faradism may succeed. In resistant cases removal of a portion of the tendon sheath is indicated. Occasionally, removal of the distal inch of the ulna becomes necessary. The triangular fibro-cartilage between the ulnar styloid process and the carpus suffers contusion, or may even be torn, and derangement can occur. Its removal may be necessary if recurring subluxation occurs.

Fractures

Obviously, if both bones are broken this is serious for a professional sportsman, as it means being off for at least three months. Even then some fractures take a much longer time to consolidate. For this reason open reduction and internal fixation should be considered. The shaft of the ulna in the forearm is amenable to a Rush or Küntscher nail introduced from the olecranon downwards, and accompanied by bone slivers taken from the

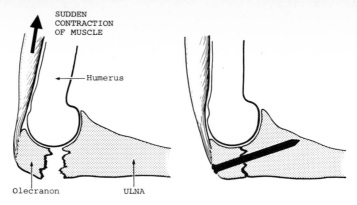

Figure 61. Treatment of fracture of right olecranon caused by strong muscular contraction of triceps: screw fixation placed obliquely.

ilium or spine of the scapula if necessary. The radius may have to be plated with special Hicks plates. Phemister bone slivers should be considered at the same time.

If conservative treatment in a plaster cast is decided upon, X-rays of the injured forearm must be compared with those of the opposite forearm taken in four planes. This comparison will demonstrate the exact amount of pronation and supination in which the arm should be placed in the plaster cast.

Fractures of the olecranon can be treated by nailing with a cancellous screw nail placed obliquely across the olecranon into the substance of the ulna distal to the coronoid process.

THE ELBOW JOINT

The elbow joint is a ginglymus composite joint consisting of:

(a) *The humero-ulnar joint*: movements of flexion and extension. Joint play movements, consisting of slight medial and lateral shift, are possible at 70° of flexion.

(b) *The humero-radial joint*: flexion and extension. Slight joint play movements in an anterior-posterior direction possible at 70° flexion as well as slight sideways movement, to what the osteopaths call 'spanning the joint', both medially and laterally. Total degree of flexion/extension movement in these joints is from 0–150°. In some elbows, hyperextension is from 10–15°, extension being 0°.

(c) *The superior radio-ulnar joint*: pronation and supination. From the neutral position between pronation and supination there is 90° of both

184

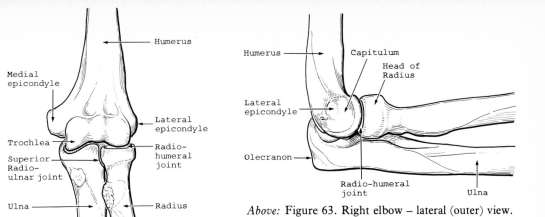

Above: Figure 62. Front view of right elbow.

Above: Figure 63. Right elbow – lateral (outer) view.

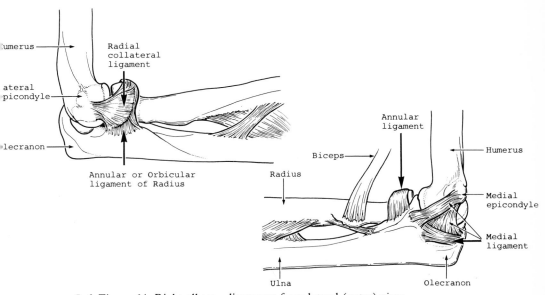

Left Figure 64. Right elbow – ligaments from lateral (outer) view.
Right: Figure 65. Right elbow – medial (inner) view. Ligaments and biceps, tendon of insertion.

movements. The various parts of the articular bony surfaces of each joint can be severally involved in different types of injury. The bony structures involved are in the humerus at the elbow joint, involving particularly the lateral epicondyle and capitellar regions, especially in young Little League baseball players; and the radial head in stress fractures and osteochondritis. Osteochondritis can be seen to affect the articular surfaces of all these

185

bones, particularly those of the radial head and the capitellum, and the opposing surfaces of the olecranon and coronoid fossae of the humerus. Also stress fractures can involve the top of the olecranon of the ulna and the head of the radius.

Synovial structures involved include the fibrous capsule structures, particularly the lateral and medial collateral, the radio-humeral collateral and orbicular ligaments.

Muscles involved are: the biceps and brachialis in front; the triceps and anconeus at the back; the extensor-supinator group on the lateral side; the flexor-pronator group on the medial side.

Certain bursae which can be involved are: (a) Osgood's Bursa on the lateral aspect. If present, it is involved in certain types of tennis elbow; (b) occasional bursae on the medial aspect between the origin of the flexors and pronators and the bone; and (c) the olecranon bursa.

INJURIES TO THE ELBOW

Sprains, strains, subluxations and dislocations of the elbow joints are notorious for slow recovery, and when the injury is of any severity many surgeons advise complete rest for a long period, usually six to eight weeks. The elbow is usually put in a plaster cast, fixed at a right angle, and gentle progressive exercises should be done without any physiotherapy. This is through fear of stimulating myositis ossificans (bony outgrowths) in the joint capsule or in the surrounding muscles, particularly in the biceps and brachialis anticus where they pass over the front of the joint. If treated by this method full flexion and extension is rarely recovered, and it may take up to one year to obtain a useful result.

Provided there is no fracture, the best way to treat elbow injuries of any severity is to place them in a removable plaster of Paris cast, split in front for ease of removal. Contrast baths, gentle exercises, short-wave, ultrasound and faradic contractions should be given the next day, and often complete recovery of full movement occurs within three weeks. In cases where there has been a subluxation or dislocation and there is marked swelling of the joint, removal of the traumatic effusion by aspiration, or Hilton's method of small incisions and insertion of sinus forceps, saves days of treatment by removing tension on the venous side of the circulation, which may be caused by the size of the traumatic effusion, which may include blood. This is essential if the swelling is interfering

186

with the circulation, in which there is a chance of Volkmann's ischaemic contracture resulting if the tension is not relieved.

In minor degrees, support by gamgee and a crêpe bandage may be sufficient.

After reduction, the stability of the joint is tested and, if found unstable, a plaster cast is applied and left on for four weeks. During this period isometric exercises are carried out three times daily, and the muscles are stimulated by faradism.

When four weeks have elapsed and the plaster of Paris is split the movements are found to be remarkably free, and physiotherapy is started daily consisting of short-wave, ultrasound and graduated movements. Full movement should be obtained in a further four weeks, but the sportsman should not return to his full sporting activities for four months at the earliest.

Strains and Sprains

Strain of muscles at their attachment to the bone is called enthesis, and occurs in cases of 'tennis elbow' and 'golf elbow'. During vigorous activity the extensor and flexor muscle attachments are strained, or even torn from their origin, either from the lateral or medial condyles. If the condition of strain persists, the underlying joint structures such as the ligaments from which the muscle fibres take origin become involved. If the strain condition persists longer, the synovial membrane and articular cartilages of the joint also may become involved, and eventually osteochondritis and osteoarthritis of the elbow, humero-radial and superior radio-ulnar joints may occur.

Tennis Elbow

Many authorities try to make out that there are many types of tennis elbow. Primarily, it is a strain or tear of the extensor muscular origins from the lateral side of the elbow, at the lateral epicondyle and the lateral humero-radial ligament. The superior radio-ulnar and humero-radial joints become involved in time if the movement of supination is added to the action of the strain. A strain or sprain occurs when the backhand stroke is performed, with the elbow in flexion.

The ideal backhand tennis stroke must be produced with the arm fully pronated (palm down), and the elbow fully extended. Bernhang has carried out extensive and important research into the tennis elbow and has

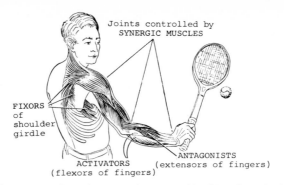

Figure 66. To demonstrate how the correctly executed backhand tennis shot is performed by activators acting in conjunction with synergists and prime fixors. At the point of impact with the ball, Pernheng has discovered that the elbow should be extended fully with the hand in the pronated position. The rest of the movement is done by the shoulder girdle and neck muscles. Often the long head of biceps is involved in front of the shoulder.

found that at the moment of impact of ball on racquet the elbow must be fully extended, and the forearm fully pronated. The rest of the movement should be performed with the elbow held straight and fully pronated. The rest of the movement should be performed by the main supinators, which are the biceps, the shoulder and the shoulder girdle muscles. Hence the almost constant involvement of the long head of biceps.

In some cases the extensor carpi radialis brevis tendon in the forearm takes origin from a fibrous band extending from the lateral humeral condyle to the tubercle of the radius. In tennis elbow this muscle is often tight, and a constant strain is thrown on this band so that it thickens and subsequently compresses the dorsal interosseus nerve in the back of the forearm, giving rise to a type of painful entrapment neuritis. This gives pain down the back of the forearm to the back of the fingers and causes weakness of this muscle.

Occasionally, in the vicinity of the origin of the extensor muscles there is a bursa (Osgood's Bursa) between the ligaments and the muscle fibres, and this may also become inflamed if present.

If the strain condition has persisted for a long time, say several months, the periosteum of the lateral epicondyle is stimulated to produce a small periosteal outgrowth, in the same way as a spur may form on the tuberosity of the os calcis (heel bone) from strain of the short muscles of the foot.

188

Although some cases of tennis elbow may be associated with a bursitis, periostitis, entrapment neuritis of the dorsal interosseus nerve and fibrillation of the head of the radius, fundamentally the basic pathology is a tear or strain of the extensor and supinator group of muscles, which may be of acute or gradual onset from progressive strain. The main flexor and supinator of the elbow joint is the biceps brachii muscle, and this muscle is very active in the backhand shot because it fixes the elbow, while at the same time it supinates the forearm. Thus the long head of biceps muscle is often involved in the tennis elbow process, as shown by tenderness of the tendon in the bicipital groove, situated in front of the shoulder joint.

As in all injuries to a part of an extremity, remedial exercises must be carried out to the muscles and joints of the whole extremity, as the effect of the injury often involves the other muscles and joints secondarily. In the case of tennis elbow, therefore, exercises must be given to the fingers, wrist, elbow, shoulder, shoulder girdle and cervical joints, of the injured side, so as to make sure that the muscles of this extremity are strengthened and returned to full power.

IMMEDIATE TREATMENT

An injection of xylocaine one per cent 5 ml with Depomedrone 1 ml is given into the tender points over the lateral epicondyle, and is combined with massage, ultrasound, wax baths and manipulations. These physical treatments should be carried out daily. The injection may have to be repeated at weekly intervals for a month. However, a vigorous regime of combined home treatment and physiotherapy will usually cure the condition in a week after one injection.

EXAMPLE

A famous Wimbledon champion developed a typical severe degree of tennis elbow three days before Wimbledon commenced. It was very acute, and it was going to be impossible for her to play unless a complete cure was obtained. On the Friday before Wimbledon she was given physiotherapy and an injection of xylocaine and Depomedrone, from which she had a violent reaction that night which lasted for twenty-four hours. She had two physiotherapy treatments on the Saturday and Sunday, with several home treatments in between, and by the Sunday evening there was a vast improvement. Luckily, the weather was so bad that she was not required to play until the following Thursday, exactly six days after the first

189

consultation. By this time the elbow and forearm were completely symptom-free, even whilst playing a strenuous match.

Occasionally, about five per cent of cases are very resistant to conservative treatment. They may require De Goes' operative removal of a pannus of synovial thickening from the humero-radial joint (called the humeral meniscus by De Goes), with release of the origin of the extensor muscles from the lateral epicondyle. Before operation, a manipulation under anaesthetic should be tried, to free adhesions and convert a tight joint into a more mobile one. Sometimes the patient has a gouty diathesis, and this should be investigated. Bernhang found that about ten per cent required operation in his series. Garden's lengthening of the extensor carpi radialis brevior in the forearm gives variable results. The prevention of strains, tears and sprains has been worked out by Bernhang in detail.

The following factors must be considered in preventing recurrences of elbow strains. In tennis these are: the weight of the racquet; the tension of the strings and what they are made of; the size of the handle; the anatomy of the tennis shot – the racquet must be held loosely at the top of the stroke and firmly just before impact with the ball. The shoulder girdle must be firmly fixed to the cervical spine and chest wall. To reiterate, in the backhand shot the time of impact with the ball should be with the elbow straight and fully pronated (palm down). After impact the forearm is supinated by the spinators (supinator brevis and biceps brachii) and abducted by the synchronous action of the shoulder girdle and shoulder girdle muscles held firmly to the neck and dorsal spine.

The Flexor-Pronator Strain – Golfing Elbow
In this condition the flexor and pronator group of muscles which are on the opposite side to that of the tennis elbow are involved on its inner side. At the beginning of the century they used to be involved in the tennis player when the forearm shot was executed with the head of the racquet dropped, and a strong spin was imparted to the ball by the action of forcibly flexing and pronating the forearm. They occur frequently in golfers and can be mild, moderate or severe, and they start in the same way as a simple muscle strain or tear which in time progresses to a joint strain and can eventually lead to osteoarthritis. Bursae, periosteal thickenings or calcareous bodies (calcium deposits) may form in relation to the capsule of the joint on the inner aspect, and delay recovery.

The right-handed golfer will sometimes suffer a type of 'tennis elbow' on the left elbow, the opposite elbow, because the follow-through of his stroke will produce strain on the extensors and supinators of this elbow. Also the right-handed golfer frequently experiences pain and loss of power in relation to the inner side of the left wrist where the triangular fibro-cartilage of the wrist, the inferior radio-ulnar joint and the extensor and flexor carpi ulnaris are involved. Strain of these structures is produced by the golf club head hitting hard ground in the act of following through with a shot.

Chondro-epiphysitis of the growing epiphyses, both on the inner aspect and the capitellar surface of the humerus, is common in the young from six to sixteen years, especially as a result of pitching at baseball.

In the act of throwing the javelin, two types of injury may be encountered. The first affects the inner side of the elbow, as in 'golfing elbow', and is due to carrying out the throw badly with a round-arm action, putting severe strain on the flexors and pronators.

The second is a stress or fatigue fracture of the tip of the olecranon from the strenuous contraction of the triceps tendon of insertion in the act of straightening the elbow when the throwing action is performed correctly. Cartilaginous loose bodies occasionally form in the elbow as the result of constant jarring of the joint surfaces, as in boxers, and, if locking occurs, they require operative removal.

THE SHOULDER JOINT

Many injuries to the shoulder joint appear trivial at first, but if left untreated will later tend to become chronic and difficult to make completely symptom-free quickly.

The total abduction movement (raising sideways) of the shoulder joint is the combined amount of the gleno-humeral and scapulo-thoracic, which is 180°. With the scapula fixed the amount of gleno-humeral movement is 90°.

If elementary anatomical studies are made of the shoulder joint, it is easy to understand the reasons why certain injuries are liable to be difficult to make symptom-free quickly. The articular surface of the head of the humerus faces that of the articular surface of the glenoid of the scapula and they are loosely held together by a capsule, which is extremely loose, particularly below and, to a lesser extent, at the back. The capsule in front is strengthened by ligaments and strong muscles which also protect the

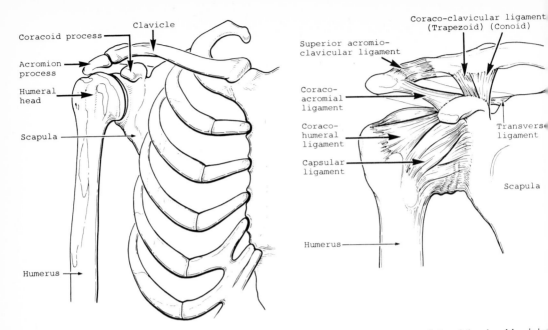

Figure 67. Right shoulder and right side of chest.　　Figure 68. Ligaments of the right shoulder join[ ]

head of the humerus in front – the subscapularis, the short head of biceps and coraco-brachialis with the latissimus dorsi. On the outer upper surface, the rotator cuff tendons, particularly the supraspinatus, and to a lesser extent the infraspinatus and teres minor, contract in action and fix and steady the head of the humerus, so that the deltoid can abduct the arm from the side. Before the deltoid muscle can take the arm outwards from the side, the head of the humerus must be steadied and fixed, thus allowing the arm to be abducted to 90°. If the palm of the hand is placed downwards in 90° abduction, the head of the humerus and the lateral part of the greater tuberosity become blocked by the acromion process of the scapula. However, when the palm of the hand is turned facing upwards in supination, the head of the humerus can now pass under the acromion process into full abduction. This is helped by the scapula rotating so that its inferior angle moves outwards and forwards. Abduction can then take place through 180° until the arm is along the side of the head.

Placed between the under surface of the deltoid muscle and the outer

192

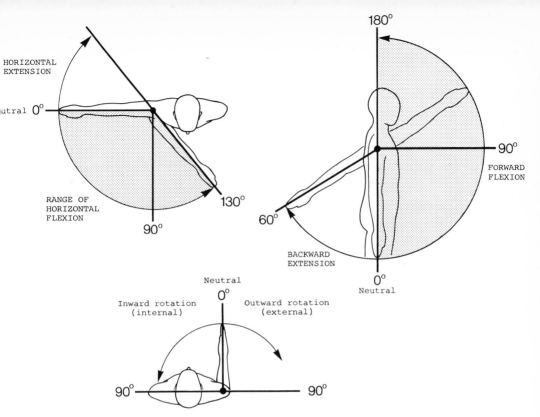

Left: Figure 69. The range of horizontal flexion and extension of the arm. *Right:* Figure 70. Motion of the arm at the shoulder vertical plane showing backward extension and forward flexion. *Centre:* Figure 71. Internal and external rotation of the arm.

side of the greater tuberosity with its attached rotated tendons is the subacromial bursa. The long head of biceps as a tendon runs from over the head of the humerus from its origin at the top of the glenoid cavity through the front of the joint and out through a groove between the two tubercles.

Injuries, especially indirect ones such as caused by throwing a ball, a weight, or discus, puts strain on any of these tendinous structures, particularly the supraspinatus and long head of biceps. They are strained, torn or ruptured, according to the severity of the injury and the subacromial bursa being placed between the deltoid muscle, and bony structures may become pinched, damaged and inflamed.

In the various positions of the head of the humerus, there must, for all movements to take place without pain, be no pathological lesions present which can obstruct movement. For example, when the abducted arm is placed as far backwards as possible, the head of the humerus travels forwards and any constricting structure such as a tight capsule, or abnormalities involving the long head of biceps, prevents this. With the arm in a forward direction the head of the humerus passes backwards. With the arm across the chest, the head of the humerus travels outwards and backwards; with the arm in abduction so that the arm rests alongside the head and neck, the head of the humerus is downwards in the glenoid. In the arm-up-the-back movement, the head of the humerus must be able to travel first forwards, then rotate fully inwards and finally travel outwards and backwards.

For full movements of the shoulder joints, not only must there be a supple capsule, but the overlying muscles must be resilient. Therefore:

1. In abducting the arm fully to lie at the side of the neck and head, the muscles of the quadrilateral space must be completely resilient. These muscles are pectoralis major and minor with the latissimus dorsi in front medially, and the triceps, teres major and minor at the back posteriorly, with the head of the humerus above and the rib cage below.

2. In adducting across the chest at the nose level, the point of the elbow must be able to line to the opposite ear.

3. In the arm-up-the-back movement, which is a composite movement of backward extension, when the head of the humerus comes forward, then the arm medially rotates and finally adducts across the back of the chest, the fingers of the opposite arm, placed above the clavicle of the same side, should be able to touch those of the arm up the back. Some sports-

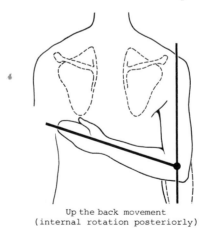

Up the back movement
(internal rotation posteriorly)

Figure 72. The first extension of the shoulder, the inward rotation and adduction. The head of the humerous first goes forwards, then inwards and finally outwards.

194

men have well developed shoulder muscles so that this is impossible, especially with the right arm up the back.

In strains or minor tears of the supraspinatus tendons, there is a painful arc in abduction between 80° and 120° due to swelling of the tendonous insertions impinging on the under surface of the acromial process. Further abduction may be painless because the tender swelling of the tendon has passed under the acromial process and pressure on it has been relieved.

Injuries either direct or indirect will cause an outpouring of traumatic effusion and blood which will quickly congeal unless dispersed and absorbed. The result is often an adherent capsulitis with adhesions in which the tendons and the subacromial bursa all become involved, by tending to stick to the head of the humerus.

Even in fractures around the shoulder joint, Perkins advocated active movements, obviously gentle at first, supporting the weight of the arm with the other hand under the point of the elbow of the injured arm, or on a pillow. If combined with physiotherapy, specially graduated faradic contractions, ultrasound, short-wave, and massage and injections of xylocaine 5 mls of one per cent with 1 or 2 mls of Depomedrone into either the supraspinatus or long head of biceps tendons, or both, at intervals, it is rewarding how quickly full recovery takes place.

Dislocations

The shoulder joint is a shallow ball-and-socket joint. The capsule and ligaments are liable through injury to become stretched, with wasting and atonia of the muscles. Because of the general laxity of shoulder joint capsule, subluxation and dislocation are not uncommon and can become recurrent. Operative reconstruction may, after three complete recurrences, be the only method making it possible for a sportsman to become active in his sport once again.

Naturally, after dislocation, reduction, often under full general anaesthesia, must be carried out, after which the head of the humerus is protected by gamgee and crêpe bandage. A check X-ray is taken. Ice-packs and isometric movements are given twice a day as well. However, the protective gamgee and bandage are removed for home treatment and physiotherapy twice daily which is given with the elbow well supported on a pillow. Radiographic control must exclude fractures of the greater

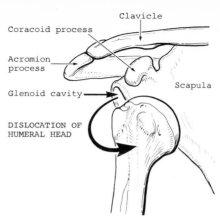

Figure 73. Dislocation of right shoulder with head displacing downwards and forwards.

tuberosity. However, the treatment is the same unless there is gross separation of fragments.

After dislocations, abduction of the arm only in a line in front of the horizontal up to a right angle is allowed for the first three weeks. Full movement should be complete in six weeks. The dislocation will recur if the lesion described by Bankart has taken place at the first injury. This lesion consists of a stripping of the capsular attachment at the front and the lower aspect of the glenoid rim and sometimes separation of a small fragment of bone from the under surface of the glenoid. Once this has occurred, no amount of rest will allow the capsule to become so firmly attached that recurrence will not take place.

It is usual to give the sportsman three separate dislocations before deciding on the need for a reconstructive operation to prevent this. However, if the sportsman is, say, a professional footballer, and the dislocation occurs in the middle of March, it will take six weeks before he can think of playing again, that is to say, not before the end of April, which really means that he should not risk playing again during that season. At this stage it is important for him to have an arthrogram of the shoulder with air and contrast media by an orthopaedic surgeon or radiologist conversant in the technique, so as to ascertain whether a Bankart lesion is present. If one is present it would be wise for him to undergo a reconstruction operation, so that by the end of August he would be fit to play again without the chance of a recurrence. Whether he has the operation or not, he should invariably wear a special check strap until he has regained confidence and full strength of the shoulder muscles.

196

Recently, a doctor, who had had a recurrent dislocation of the shoulder joint operated on without success, was seen in consultation. He was captain of his hospital rugby side and wanted to continue to lead his side in the hospital cup-ties. He managed to do this successfully wearing one of the check straps without buckles but held together by velcro bands. It is most uncommon for recurrence to take place after a reconstruction has been properly performed.

Severe Sprain

If, after injury, the sportsman cannot abduct the arm at all, it is possible that rupture of the supraspinatus tendon has taken place. If the AT Approach is adopted it is surprising how some of these cases show recovery in a few days, but if there is no evidence of this after ten days, operation should be considered. An arthrograph often helps. Occasionally the tendon of insertion into the greater trochanter is avulsed with a fragment of bone and these cases require immediate replacement of the tendon and, if necessary, should be held firmly with a small screw or staple.

Sub-acute and Chronic Sprains and Capsulitis (Frozen Shoulder)

If a painful shoulder is seen six or more weeks after injury, examination may reveal limitation of abduction and other movements of varying degrees. Painful tender points are found over long head of biceps in its groove and specially in relation to the sub-deltoid bursa and supraspinatus tendon of insertion. Radiographs may reveal a plague of ossification in relation to the tendon or the bursa.

Probably in this type of case it is wise to give two injections of xylocaine and Depomedrone at three-day intervals with vigorous home treatment and physiotherapy and observe if there is any improvement. If this is marked, continuation on the same line is indicated; manipulation under anaesthetic is only advised when improvement stops. However, if there is no improvement from the start after the first injection and two days of treatment, manipulation under anaesthesia may be the quickest way to complete recovery. The mistake of over-manipulating must not be made. If a case is markedly limited in movement, it may be wise to carry out the manipulation under anaesthesia in two stages, gaining a certain degree at the first, which is completed a month later after further home treatment and physiotherapy.

MANIPULATION OF THE SHOULDER UNDER AN ANAESTHETIC

It is imperative to be certain that the manipulation is going to take place when the condition of capsulitis is in the positive healing phase. If the manipulation is carried out in the negative phase exacerbation of the condition is certain with increase of symptoms. The correct method of ascertaining in which stage the condition is present is to treat the patient for a few days and be sure that there is slight improvement after each treatment. After the manipulation 20 mls one per cent xylocaine with 2 mls Depomedrone are injected into the tissue when it is considered that adhesions have broken. Frequent physiotherapy, daily if possible, should be given afterwards, particularly gentle progressive mani-pulations, otherwise there is a tendency for the joint to freeze again.

During this period it is wise to support the elbow in a universal sling (see Figure 75), taking it out several times each day for exercises.

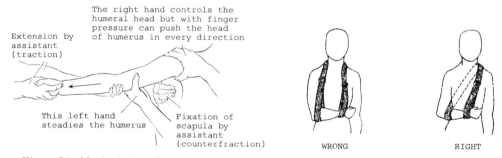

Figure 74. Manipulation of the shoulder joint.

Figure 75. Universal sling. It is essential *not* have sling suspended from around neck b from opposite shoulder.

Occasionally one sees an older athlete who gives a history of previous shoulder injury and disability. In most cases, he has experienced occa-sional twinges of pain on certain movements, such as bringing the arm up suddenly in the abducted, horizontal, extended position. He comes in with excruciating pain, which prevents sleep, and most movements are moderately limited. X-rays may show calcification in the tendon of the supraspinatus or sub-acromial bursa. If an injection of xylocaine and Depomedrone does not alleviate the excruciating pain within twenty-four

198

hours, operation under general anaesthesia to release the calcium deposit is indicated. Occasionally this calcium deposit is under such tension that it will shoot up under pressure, hitting the ceiling of the operating theatre. This is not an exaggeration, for the tension which these deposits of calcium are under accounts for the severe pain.

Once an injured shoulder has been allowed to become chronic, it can be extremely difficult to make symptom-free quickly. An example of this difficulty was shown in the case of a famous bowler who, six years ago, was unable to complete the cricket season because of pain when trying to bowl. He also suffered a constant ache in the shoulder and, in his case, X-rays of the shoulder and cervical spine were normal, but he had limitation of the extremes of all movements as well as tender areas in relation to the long head of biceps and rotator cuff insertions. There was a history of trouble with his shoulder in previous cricket seasons and in this one he broke down towards the end of the season and was unable to carry on.

He was diagnosed as having a recurring rotator cuff and long head of biceps strain with a general sprain of the joint. These gave rise to limitation of movement due to capsular adhesions and thickenings on the tendons, with contraction of the surrounding muscles, thus limiting their full movements.

Before he became symptom-free he required a great deal of daily treatment, starting with two injections of xylocaine and Depomedrone. In addition, at the end of a week's treatment he was given a manipulation under anaesthesia to ensure full range of movement, but before he bowled again freely he required home treatment twice daily and physiotherapy five times weekly for three months. No doubt he was the type of case on whom many surgeons would have advised operative treatment, and this would have been necessary if he had not recovered by the beginning of January, treatment having been commenced at the end of the cricket season. This same player bowled successfully for five seasons, but in the middle of a recent season sustained a severe contusion sprain of the same shoulder in falling whilst fielding a ball. In this injury he stretched and caused neurapraxia (concussion injury) to the long nerve of Bell, which supplies the rhomboid muscles and the serratus anticus muscles. The result was a slight winging of the scapula and although he had daily treatment with support to the shoulder girdle, he was out of cricket for eight weeks.

Sometimes operative procedures are considered to be a quicker and

199

more certain method of making these cases symptom-free. Three types of operation have been described to cover resistant cases. The first, acromiectomy (Watson Jones), is not a good operation because the recovery time is sometimes up to a year. The second, described by Stamm, is osteotomy of the glenoid neck which allows the head of the humerus to drop thus permitting the structures inserted into the greater tuberosity to pass freely under the acromion process in abduction. He found this out in a patient who was suffering intense pain and inability to abduct the arm until she fell and fractured the neck of the glenoid. Immediate improvement followed. As a result of this he tried this operation out on a series of patients with similar symptoms, with good results. The third operation, described by Carter Rowe, is designed to flatten the greater tuberosity, at the same time incising and removing a section of the coraco-acromial ligament. This ligament is inclined in most cases to be thickened, which prevents the free passage of the greater tuberosity to travel through to full abduction of the arm. With the removal of some of the greater tuberosity by flattening it and sectioning the ligament, the obstructing factors are removed. This operation would appear to be the easiest of the three and gives good, relatively quick results.

FRACTURES OF THE CLAVICLE

These are relatively frequent fractures in all sports, as falls on the shoulder occur often. They are treated mostly by a figure-of-eight bandage and sling, neither of which controls the fracture. Usually, in any type of fracture of the clavicle, there is involvement of the neck and shoulder muscles as strains or tears, and it is these that often give rise to pain and disability later unless treated from the first. It is common to see a traumatic capsulitis of the shoulder with limited neck movements some five weeks after a badly treated fracture of the clavicle. Some authorities think that a simple sling is sufficient support to jockeys who want to return to riding quickly under stress.

It has been found that the use of clavicle rings with a pad and strapping over the fracture site gives excellent results, especially if a check brace is applied to the clavicle rings at the back. They brace the shoulders outwards. The check brace, which can be made of stockinet, is brought forwards round the front of the rib cage and periodically tightened. This has the benefit of easy adjustment, removal for baths and physiotherapy to

200

the shoulder and neck muscles, at the same time keeping the shoulder well braced back. The bracing-back of the shoulders is supplemented by a universal sling, which has a fixed loop round the elbow and a loose adjustable strap which goes up the back and over the uninjured shoulder, where the support of the injured arm is taken, instead of around the neck. This also helps to keep the shoulders braced well back.

EXAMPLE 1

A famous flat-race jockey sustained a fall, causing a simple non-displaced fracture of the left clavicle. The important point with regard to recovery was that at the same time he sprained his left shoulder and cervical vertebral joints, so that there was marked tenderness of the neck and shoulder muscles, with almost complete loss of movement of the left shoulder and cervical vertebral joints. He was treated at first with a protection pad and waterproof strapping over the site of the fracture. Clavicle rings and a universal sling to keep the shoulder braced backwards lessened the strain on the clavicle at the fracture site. He was able to carry out remedial exercises and home treatment with physiotherapy as by the AT Approach. On the seventh day there was some tenderness over the long head of biceps in its groove in front of the left shoulder, and an injection of xylocaine and Depomedrone was given. He was encouraged to ride and, after the injection that day, he found he could do so without any undue symptoms. On exactly the eleventh day after injury he won two races consecutively at Epsom without any untoward ill effects. If he had been a footballer this quick return to his sport would have been impossible.

Provided there is good protection to the brachial vessels and nerves by an intact inner two-thirds of the clavicle, fractures at the junction of the outer third can be treated quickly and successfully by removing it. Fractures treated in this way have enabled a rider to return to full activities of competitive riding within ten days.

EXAMPLE 2

A show jumper fractured his left clavicle at the junction of the inner two-thirds with the outer third. The outer third was removed, and while the stitches were still *in situ* on the fourth day he practised jumping hurdles. The stitches were removed on the seventh day, and on the tenth day he took part in competitions, winning a first and two seconds.

EXAMPLE 3

Another jockey had both outer ends of clavicle removed for fractures. He

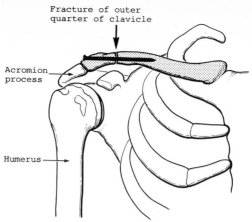

Figure 76. Fracture of right clavicle treated by screw fixation.

was then known as 'the boneless Hercules', as his shoulders were so strong!

Some surgeons prefer to immobilise the fracture with a suitable screw, especially when there is gross overlapping of the fragments. However, firm immobilisation by clavicle rings and a universal sling is essential after the operation for two months to allow consolidation of the fracture. Most athletes prefer other methods.

SUBLUXATION OF THE ACROMIO-CLAVICULAR JOINT

This joint is a common site of injury, as falling on the shoulder is a frequent occurrence in every type of sport. Unless there is complete dislocation, an Active Therapeutic Approach is started immediately with injection of one per cent xylocaine 2 ml with Depomedrone 1 ml into the joint. Sometimes, after the xylocaine is injected and before the Depomedrone is instilled, aspiration of bloody synovial fluid should take place if present. This lessens swelling, and with a padded support over the joint held in position with clavicle rings, and the arm supported in a universal sling, the degree of subluxation usually rapidly returns to nearly normal.

In most cases there has been a sprain of the shoulder joint and the cervical vertebral joints as well, with involvement of the overlying muscles, and if they are not included in the treatment, thickenings and adhesions in these joints will form and retard recovery, possibly for many months. Some authorities advise immediate operation in these cases of subluxation, but often recurrence takes place after the operation on the

202

first occasion that the sportsman falls on his shoulder. If treatment is carried out so that the products of contused, bruised tissues around the joint itself and the shoulder and neck muscles are removed quickly, the patient can often return to vigorous exercise within a month.

Some subluxations have been allowed to become chronic, and, if left long enough, osteoarthritis will have set in. Removal of the outer one inch of the clavicle often gives a painless result in a short time, especially if, after operation, rehabilitation of the shoulder, scapular and neck muscles are carried out soon.

DISLOCATION OF THE ACROMIO-CLAVICULAR JOINT
A complete dislocation in an athlete can be most disabling. If operation is decided upon, grafting the upper third of the coracoid with the origin of the long head of biceps and coraco-brachialis muscles attached is proving to be the most satisfactory and permanent method. This graft is attached by strong silk or wire sutures to the front and lower surfaces of the outer end of the clavicle, and the joint capsule reconstructed with a part of the acromio-clavicular ligament. Following operation, a firm pressure pad is worn for five weeks. The transplanted biceps and coraco-brachialis muscles now attached to the outer end of the clavicle help to hold it down in position.

Another alternative which gives a quicker result is to remove the outer inch of the clavicle.

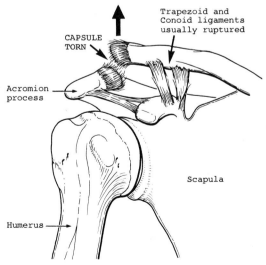

Figure 77. Dislocation of right acromio-clavicular joint.

203

The Difficult Case and Conclusions

Some cases are difficult to get right quickly by conservative methods and these include: shoulder sprains, particularly in the older sportsman; certain cases of tenosynovitis (tendons); cases of chondromalacia patellae (knee); osteochondritis (inflammation of articular cartilage of the joints); some contusions and sprains of carpal and tarsal joints (wrist and foot).

The presence of a septic, toxic or gouty diathesis must be excluded as well as the presence of a 'tight joint'. Some joints are tight from birth due to a congenital abnormality such as a short ilio-psoas (groin) muscle. Others become tight through injury and inflammation.

In some cases operation may be the quickest method. However, often a series of injections combined with home treatment and physiotherapy over three or four weeks will produce signs of improvement sufficient to justify continuing with conservative treatment until full recovery is obtained.

If a painful injured joint or contused bone still has symptoms two months after injury, further X-rays and blood tests may be advisable. Once a bone is contused it will not become symptom-free until all the products of bruising have been dispersed. Manipulation under a general anaesthetic, combined with injections, or even operation may be necessary to obtain a quicker result.

There are conditions in which the experienced surgeon will consider that operative measures will remove the products of injury such as haematoma and necrotic tissue by the stroke of the knife. The surgeon can also by surgical means overcome quickly the effects of injury such as would occur in a dislocation of a joint, for example the shoulder. In such case an arthrogram may reveal that the sportsman has a typical lesion in which recurrence is likely and an immediate operation is more certain as it will allow return to full activity within four months for cricket and golf, and six months for more violent sports.

In the early 1950s the Southampton Football Club worked on the slogan 'Treat and Train' and this should be the motto of any sports injury clinic. After the Second World War sports clinics multiplied, but only minimally in this country compared to Europe and the USA.

Few national sports organise early treatment in sports clinics for their participants, but there are several exceptions to this. For example, the British Amateur Boxing Association, through the work of Dr J. L.

Blonstein OBE, has made it a rule for a doctor to be present at every boxing match in the country.

Most professional soccer teams have a medical set-up, but the poorer ones depend on hospitals, where if the injured player has a sprained ankle he is X-rayed and, if this proves negative, he is told he has sprained his ankle and is given a bandage, usually without instructions about the type and amount of exercise he should carry out. He is told to return in a week, by which time the ankle is even more painful and the movements are becoming restricted.

Sometimes injured joints are strapped up at once so that when swelling occurs in the night the patient suffers great pain. A firm crêpe bandage over cottonwool allows for swelling and can be taken off easily for contrast baths and physiotherapy. It should be a general rule never to strap injuries immediately after their occurrence, but support them with a split plaster cast or gamjee and crêpe bandages.

When the sportsman plays his first game after injury, strapping support may then be indicated. Some injured joints may swell during treatment and this reaction may even help absorb the products of injury. If excessive swelling takes place, a short period of rest from exercise may be indicated but contrast baths and physiotherapy must be continued.

If a case is not improving, the surgeon should review the history of injury and physical signs and symptoms and should remember to check on the patient's blood to rule out the possibility of a toxic focus or metabolic diathesis, such as gout.

If a footballer has a fractured wrist and it is in a plaster cast he can, while the fracture is mending, endeavour to make his kicking more efficient. In football this has happened in the case of several well-known players who, during their period of rehabilitation for fractures of the upper extremity, have made themselves proficient at kicking goals.

The surgeon will usually obtain the full co-operation of the injured sportsman by explaining the exact nature of his injury. He will then carry out every detail of the AT Approach and never miss a chance of rehabilitating himself to his full sporting activities.

The injured sportsman should supply sixty per cent improvement to his injury whereas the medical profession divided between the surgeon, physiotherapist and trainer requires only to supply forty per cent. If the sportsman only supplies thirty per cent by inefficient home treatment, but the medical side accomplishes its full forty per cent, the total is then only seventy per cent improvement, which is not sufficient to make everyday life free from symptoms, as eighty per cent improvement is required for normal everyday exercise; ninety per cent is required for moderate exercises and one hundred per cent for full vigorous functions.

Unless a joint has recovered one hundred per cent of its movement and muscle power it is liable to have a return of symptoms. This criterion is often well understood by lay practitioners who have been taught the methods of joint manipulation, and accounts for their successes.

Throughout the programme of AT Approach the injured sportsman is being continuously motivated to becoming one-hundred-per-cent fit. This is relatively easy as he is usually dedicated to his particular sport. He must be encouraged to carry out his home treatment with Vim and Vigour, Religiously, Regularly, Resolutely, Reasonably – if somewhat Reluctantly. Stress is made that Practice and Perseverance of Physical Principles Promotes Perfect Posture.

5
Rehabilitation before Retraining

Even though an injury has been successfully treated and the athlete pronounced fit to return to his sport, some weakness in the damaged part may remain. The aim of treatment is to get one-hundred-per-cent complete recovery. This means a full range of movement and muscle control. The joint must be as stable as it was before the injury: any residual weaknesses may result in a repetition of the accident and not necessarily under the same conditions.

For example, an ankle which has been damaged at football may, if not completely stable and rehabilitated, rick in a game of tennis or golf, in skiing or even walking along the street. Or again, a collarbone broken in a riding accident may be associated with stiffness in the shoulder and neck muscles with limitation of movement, and these can be aggravated and give rise to painful symptoms in other sports like shooting, or any sport in which the shoulder and neck are used.

After the injury the muscles and soft tissues may become contracted and shortened and lose their resilience and elasticity. If this is not successfully counteracted, the joints may also undergo deterioration, and eventually degeneration, leading later in life to osteoarthritis – though this is a situation that the young sportsman may feel is too far off to worry about. His successful return to his sport, however, is something that matters to him. *Home treatment* when done regularly and conscientiously after an accident can do more than prevent deterioration in the future. It can ensure that the sportman goes back into his sport in perfect condition.

He should learn always to stand in the Active Alerted Posture as this not only distributes the body weight evenly over the joints, and especially the joint which is recovering, but also prepares it for action and helps prevent future injury. Home treatment can be started, with the doctor's permission, even while the limb is in plaster of Paris or immobilised in some other way. Isometric exercises, elevation and hanging the limb can each be done for fifteen minutes daily, as can surging faradism if a faradic battery is available. Contrast baths can be used to bring extra blood-flow to the injured part. Products of injury are thereby carried away more rapidly.

Contrast bathing can be done in several ways, depending on the region of the injured part, beginning and ending with very hot water, as hot as it can be borne, and then alternating with ice-cold water. Two basins and two sponges can be used or a hot and then a cold shower taken. The sponge-and-basin method has the advantage that ice can be placed in the water. Two minutes of hot followed by two minutes of cold (ten minutes in all) is the correct procedure. *Always* start and finish with hot.

Self-physiotherapy is a useful adjunct to the physiotherapy that may be given in the clinic or hospital. The recovering athlete can use talcum powder or a lubricating ointment, such as Vaseline or Nivea, and gently rub the injured part, learning to dig the fingers into the tender points. He may also have a heat lamp.

Exercises in the bath are easy to do and additions to the water will help to give a special spa treatment. For instance, if coarse sea salt is added (obtainable from health stores) it gives the same effect as a dip in the ocean. The salt is good for the skin, containing, as it does, all the minerals of the sea. A seaweed preparation can be added which also contains valuable sea minerals, especially iodine, a powerful disinfectant. Liquid seaweed added to hot water helps the body to get rid of impurities through additional sweating.

The bath is a good place to do some rehabilitating and general exercises.

Bath Exercise 1: for the Shoulder Girdle

Sitting upright and with extended arms, clasp the hands in front. Keeping the arms straight, swing them overhead, then bend arms at the elbow, swing them over and clasp the back of the head, elbows pulled back. Press the head against the resisting hands, bringing the elbows forward slowly. Relax and repeat five times.

Bath Exercise 2: for the Hips and Pelvis, and also to Strengthen the Lower Spine

Lean against the back of the bath with feet pressing against the tap end. Push the feet alternately against the bath end like a cat pressing its paws on a blanket. Do this twelve times.

Bath Exercise 3: for the Lower Back

Sit upright in the bath, pull in the muscles of the abdomen slowly, starting at the pit of the stomach. Roll the muscles as if to tuck them under the ribs. Hold for a count of six and then very slowly relax. Repeat six times.

Bath Exercise 4: for the Hip Joints, Pelvis and Lower Back

Resting against the back of the bath put the legs straight out in front of you. Rest one foot on the instep of the other. Press the top foot against the resistance of the lower foot. Reverse foot. Repeat five times.

Bath Exercise 5: for the Feet and Ankles

Sitting upright in the bath, feet at a right angle to the legs, turn toes in. Pull the foot up towards the insides of the ankles. Turn the toes out and pull up to the outsides of the ankles. Do six times on each side and then repeat, but this time curling the toes and keeping them curled as you pull up. These exercises can also be done in bed.

SWIMMING

This is one of the best possible rehabilitation exercises because it is non-weight-bearing. Even if the pool is small there are exercises that can be valuable because they are done against a natural resistance of the water. Swimming uses every muscle in the body.

Non-weight-bearing means, of course, that the water bears the weight in a way that air does not. It counteracts the effects of gravity. On the other hand, air offers no resistance to the free movement of arms and legs while water does. It is this basic fact which makes water exercises different from any others.

Pool Exercise 1: for the Insides of the Thighs

Stand in the shallow end, holding on to the side of the pool. Allow the left leg to float slowly sideways to the surface until it is an near as possible at right angles to the body. Then press it down again hard, against the resistance of the water. Repeat with the right leg. (If this exercise is done on dry land the effort of bringing it up ensures that the exact opposite muscles are used.) Do this exercise six times with each leg.

Pool Exercise 2: for the Waist and Top Half of the Spine

Stand in water up to the neck with feet wide apart, arms outstretched, abdomen taut and tucked in. Twist at the waist, swinging the whole torso sideways, pressing slowly but firmly against the resistance of the water. Swing slowly and purposefully round, pushing the resisting water away

o

from you. Keep head still and eyes looking straight ahead, which gives extra resistance. Six times each side.

Pool Exercise 3: for the Knees and Circulation
Run on the spot, raising knees as high as possible. This can be done at several depths for as long as you want.

Pool Exercise 4: for the Feet
Rise on the tips of the toes ballet-style. Although this is not feasible on dry land, except, of course, for the ballet dancer, the water makes it easy by supporting the weight of the body. Walk on your 'points', at neck depth, holding the body very straight and with the head held high.

Pool Exercise 5: for the Knees and Hips
At a depth of three feet do a Russian sword dance, shooting feet vigorously out in front of you.

Pool Exercise 6: for the Hips and Legs
Using a corner of the pool at the shallow end, rest your arms on the pool's ledge and support your weight on them – the water bears most of this burden. Spread your legs out behind you and swing the left leg over the right, then the right over the left in a scissors movement. Legs should be straight out at about waist height. Repeat six times.

UNDERWATER MASSAGE
Rub, squeeze and knead the part that was injured and do those of the 'land' exercises that particularly apply to the injured part. Most of them can be adapted to water.

HOME TREATMENT AND EXERCISES FOR THE NECK
The cause of injury may be a fall in polo or any other equestrian sport; a motor racing or motor cycle racing accident could result in a break or dislocation or a whiplash injury, as could a head-on blow in rugby. A sudden whipping accident to the head in boxing may cause an injury.

A collar may have been prescribed while the injury was recovering. It is a good thing to continue to wear this at night or even intermittently during the day. A woollen muffler worn while sleeping or an electric hot pad wrapped round the neck when first in bed may help relax the muscles.

Contrast baths and self-physiotherapy also strengthen weakened muscles and help to relieve tension.

The following exercises may be done at odd moments during the day, though six times for each one is enough at any session.

Neck Exercise 1

Self-manipulation, if the doctor advises it, can be performed by rotating the neck to the right, assisted by the right hand, which should cup the chin. The left hand should first be at the back of the head near the top. Pull each hand in an opposite direction using small, jerky movements. This helps to twist the second cervical vertebra on the first. Do twelve small movements then repeat on the opposite side. Next, keeping the chin cupped, move the other hand further down the head and repeat as before. This reaches the lower vertebra. With the third movement one hand cups the chin, the other is at the back of the neck, reaching an even lower vertebra.

Neck Exercise 2

Sitting upright, chin tucked in, back of the neck straight, bend the head very slowly forward to a count of six, then very slowly backward to a count of six, six times each way.

Neck Exercise 3

In the same position turn the head as far as possible to the left to a slow count of six, then slowly to the right, keeping the back of the neck straight. Do this six times each way.

Neck Exercise 4

Grip the sides of the chair so as to fix the shoulders and then bend the head slowly to the left side, trying to touch the shoulder with the ear (but without strain). Do this to a slow count of six and similarly go over to the right. Do the double movement six times.

Neck Exercise 5

Still with fixed shoulders, rotate the head slowly clockwise then anti-clockwise (six times each way), bending the head over as far as possible.

HOME TREATMENT AND EXERCISES FOR SHOULDER GIRDLE AND COLLARBONE

Dislocations and subluxations are among the commonest injuries in many sports and in athletes. A broken clavicle – collarbone – can often happen to steeplechase jockeys, show jumpers, three-day-eventers, or in any sport in which the athlete falls on the shoulder or outstretched hand. It can also happen if a gun kicks back while game shooting. There is sometimes a subluxation of the outer or inner end of the collarbone.

On returning to active sport the injured shoulder should be well protected as otherwise the injury might be reactivated. It should be well strapped or a shoulder harness worn if allowed, or the joint protected or supported with a felt pad or strapping. Steeplechase jockeys often choose to ride at an early stage in recovery wearing clavicle rings, even running the risk of damaging their injured shoulder further rather than give up riding in an important race.

Anyone who has dislocated or subluxed a shoulder, or has had a clavicle injury, should continue his home treatment and exercises until he feels completely recovered. In addition, Active Alerted Posture should always be practised because the position in which the shoulder is held in this posture is important in preventing the weight of gravity causing degenerative changes in the shoulder and cervical spinal joints. The shoulders should always be lifted and relaxed, held slightly forward, so that the arms are not a dead weight on the shoulder girdle.

The following exercises should be done with both arms, even if only one has been injured.

Shoulder Exercise 1

With the tops of the arms close to the body, swing the arms from elbow forward, down, sideways, down, backwards, down; repeat six times.

Shoulder Exercise 2

Bending forward from the waist with the arm hanging down in front, fists facing frontwards, make six forward circles, then reverse the wrists with the fists facing backward; make six backward circles.

Shoulder Exercise 3

Bring the right hand to the shoulder. Cup the right elbow with the left hand and gently press upwards to a count of six. Repeat on the other side even if only one shoulder is painful.

HOME TREATMENT FOR THE ARMS AND ELBOWS

As is the case for all injuries, the muscles of the arm which has been involved tend to waste and must be returned to normal before the sport is resumed. The whole arm must be treated as an entity.

In tennis or golf the elbow joint and its surrounding muscles are prone to recurrent strain (this of course applies to all sports where a racquet is used), secondary to a sprain or progressive strain of the lifting muscles of the forearm. If this is not corrected the shoulder and neck muscles may become involved.

Anyone who has once had any symptoms of a 'tennis elbow' (the right-handed golfer can get it in the left elbow) should continue home treatment as long as he continues the game itself and even after, since, in an older person, the chronic 'tennis elbow' may become osteoarthritic.

The original cause may have been a continuous and prolonged incorrect use of the forearm muscles and this should be corrected before returning to play. For instance, in a backhand tennis shot the activator muscles should be aided by the synergists at wrist, elbow and shoulder, but firmly controlled by the fixors at the shoulder girdle and neck, and the whole arm, from shoulder to fingers, moved as a controlled entity.

If there has been a fracture or a dislocation of the elbow or shoulder very gentle exercises should be performed. Too-vigorous exercises or physiotherapy may cause calcification to occur in the ligaments and near the joints. There should be no lifting or carrying of heavy articles and deep massage around the elbow should never be given within the first four months after the injury.

The following four exercises are designed to put the elbow joint through its full range of movement and at the same time strengthen the associated muscles.

Elbow Exercise 1

Holding a small plastic sponge or an unrolled Elastoplast bandage, and with the arms at the sides, squeeze the bandage as you raise the arms to touch the shoulders (use both arms even if only one was injured). Return to starting position. Do this six times, squeezing the bandage on bending, relaxing when straightening, fists facing forward.

Elbow Exercise 2

Reverse the wrists so that fists face backward and repeat the exercise. Do this six times.

Elbow Exercise 3

With wrists facing forward and at shoulder height, drop the fists, still clenching the bandage. Squeeze the bandage on straightening, relax on bending six times.

Elbow Exercise 4

With wrists facing backward repeat Exercise 3 six times.

Elbow Exercise 5

Do an imaginary tennis backward shot, holding the upper arm with the other hand so that the movement is restricted to the elbow. Do this six times.

Elbow Exercise 6

This exercise is beneficial to the wrist and shoulder joints but particularly to the elbow. Sitting upright, let the arms hang at the side. Make a fist and rotate the fist and the entire arm outwards as far as possible and then right round inwards as far as possible. Rotate right out and down and then right in and down six times.

HOME TREATMENT AND EXERCISES FOR FINGERS, HANDS AND WRISTS

Hands, wrists and fingers can be damaged at almost any sport. Fingers can receive a direct blow from a ball, be trodden on in football, snapped or dislocated when they take the brunt of a fall. The complications which can occur with broken, sprained or dislocated fingers or thumbs are usually due to disturbed blood circulation: traumatic effusions of blood and lymph not being readily or fully absorbed. When this happens, adhesions and thickenings result with stiffness and limitation of movement and chronic stiffness of joints and even, eventually, deformity.

Fractures, dislocations or subluxations of the wrist are more common than anywhere else in the body as one or other of these may happen if the hand is put down to avert a fall.

Until the condition is one-hundred-per-cent symptom-free contrast baths should be given twice daily to help disperse the effusions. For a broken wrist without displacement a protective wrist gauntlet may be used fastened with Velcro for easy removal.

214

Sprains and strains of the wrist occur in sports where a racquet, club or other tool is used incorrectly over a period without the wrist being properly fixed with the balanced action of the surrounding tendons.

The following wrist exercises are designed to put the joint through a full range of movement.

Wrist Exercise 1

Rest the forearm on a table with the wrist and hand extended over the edge, palms facing down. Bend the wrist down and up six times.

Wrist Exercise 2

Same position but make a fist and rotate the wrist clockwise six times, then anti-clockwise six times.

Wrist Exercise 3

Same position but swing the hands from side to side from the wrist six times.

Wrist Exercise 4

Same position, then twist the palms upward and then downward, six times.

Finger Exercise 1

Clench the fists on a ball of foam or a rolled bandage and squeeze. Six times, both hands together.

Finger Exercise 2

'Play the piano' on the table, raising the fingers high.

Finger Exercise 3

Spread hands flat on a table top, spread fingers apart and bring them together again. Do this six times, both hands simultaneously.

Finger Exercise 4

Palms flat on the table, lift all the fingers together, extending the tips backward six times.

Finger Exercise 5

Keeping fingers flat on the table top, lift the palms six times.

Finger Exercise 6

Hands together in front of you, palms and fingers together, fingers pointing upward as in prayer. Press the fingers only over to the left keeping the palms upright and without giving way in the wrist. Press the fingers on the left hand backwards with the fingers of the right. Do this twelve times and then reverse.

Finger Exercise 7

In the same position, pull the palms away from the fingers, keeping the insides of the knuckles together, especially the little fingers. The wrists should come up at right angles. Do this twelve times.

HOME TREATMENT FOR THE SPINE AND DISCS

Injuries to the back can always be serious and, if the spinal cord has been damaged, paralysis may have occurred. A break may cause some displacement of the backbone (vertebral bodies) and no exercises should be undertaken without the approval of the doctor.

There are three levels of the spine where most strains or sprains occur: the head on the neck; the shoulder girdle and upper back; the lower back below the waist. These can result from an acute sudden movement incorrectly carried out, such as picking up a weight with the knees stiff and the back bent over. Fractures can happen in the top (cervical), mid (dorsal) and lower (lumbar) spine as a result of a fall on the feet. Any spinal injury previously experienced weakens the back muscles and makes a recurrence likely. Bowling and fielding at cricket and in many other sports may result in a damaged back.

After recovery the back may still need a support or brace, or a webbing corset, especially on returning to active sport, and attention should be given to posture, home treatment and strengthening exercises as soon as the doctor permits. In bending forward, the movement should always be against the resistance of the abdominal muscles which should actively pull the trunk forward.

Dr Hugh Bury of Guy's Hospital advocates LIFE (Lumbar Isometric Flexion Exercises). Exercises which use the muscles attaching the trunk to the pelvis and the pelvis to the thigh are needed for many months after the injury is healed. Active Alerted Posture advocates standing with the abdominal muscles pulled up and the buttocks tucked under so that the

216

back is flattened. It is from this position that one should bend forward so that the trunk and pelvis move together and the pivot takes place through the hip joint instead of at the lumbo-sacral (low back) level.

Lower Back Exercise 1
Lie flat on the floor with knees bent, spine touching the ground. Raise the head as far as possible, then down again, six times.

Lower Back Exercise 2
Lying down, arch the back with buttocks on the floor. Flatten the back by pressing the spine down. Tighten the buttocks and raise them off the floor. This is done in three distinct movements, six times.

Mid-Back Exercise 3
Sit on a stool with the feet flat on the floor, together and parallel, arms out in front, palms down. Rotate the trunk first to the right, then to the left, swinging as far possible in each direction and holding for a few seconds at each side. Repeat six times.

Mid-Back Exercise 4
Same position but hands on hips. Side-bend, first to the right then to the left, holding a few seconds at each extreme. Do this six times.

Mid-Back Exercise 5
Same position, rotate the trunk from the waist making a circle. Do this first clockwise six times then anti-clockwise six times.

HOME TREATMENT AND EXERCISES FOR HIPS AND THIGHS
When athletes fracture their thighs it is usually in the middle or lower end of the femur – the main bone that runs through the thigh. Pulled hamstring muscles – charleyhorse – and other strains and sprains of the upper leg muscles usually occur after a fast sprint. Fractures can happen in skiing, football, all equestrian sports, and in various types of athletics. Strains may be due to insufficient warm-up before running.

Dislocation of the hip is rare in athletics. It is a vulnerable area for contusions in sports where hitting a hard ground is likely: rugby football,

217

ice hockey, falls in equestrian sports. Strains of the hip muscles are common and often associated with bursitis.

It is most important to make sure there is a full range of movement after recovery before returning to active sport. This can be accomplished by graduated exercises. Kneading and massage are also useful.

Hip and Thigh Exercise 1
Lying on the back, legs out straight, feet a few inches apart, turn the toes inwards as far as they will go, then outwards as far as they will go. This rotates the hip. Repeat six times.

Hip and Thigh Exercise 2
Lying on the back, bringing one knee to the chest and circle it first clockwise, then anti-clockwise. Change legs and repeat, six times each side. Keep the back flat on the floor at the waist.

Hip and Thigh Exercise 3*
Standing upright, holding on to the back of a chair for support; start by putting all the weight on the left foot. Then raise the hip and the heel of the right foot, swing the toes in and the heel out. Do not point the foot down. With an upright posture raise the leg sideways and go on pulling the leg back and out. Repeat on the other leg. Do this twelve times, alternating legs.

Hip and Thigh Exercise 4*
The second movement is carried out in the same position holding to the back of a chair. Standing on both feet, transfer all the weight to the left foot, raise the hip and the heel on the right side and put the leg diagonally back with the foot turned out, not pointed down. Raise the leg from the hip, and go on pulling the leg up in small further movements. Do this twelve times then change legs.

Hip and Thigh Exercise 5*
The third of this series is performed in the same position. Raise the hip

* These exercises were devised by Joanna Lewis.

218

and the heel on the right side and go back with the left, upright posture –
twelve times each leg.

Hip and Thigh Exercise 6

Sitting on the floor, bend forward and grasp the toes if possible. Don't
strain if you can only reach the ankles or calves. Draw the top of the body
towards the feet, with the head as far as possible towards the knees. Hold
for a count of six and repeat six times.

HOME TREATMENT AND EXERCISES FOR THE KNEE

The knee joint, though it is surrounded by powerful muscles and strong
ligaments is, nevertheless, very vulnerable to both direct and indirect
injuries. Torn ligaments are common in many sports; ligaments are there
to stabilise the joint by preventing undue movement. The severity of the
injury often depends on how badly the ligaments are strained, torn or
ruptured.

Dislocations are uncommon although in some cases the patella – knee
cap – dislocates.

Subluxations occur from lax ligaments and lead to joint instability.

After a knee injury, especially a dislocation or subluxation, (and some
American college football team managers say before, as a preventive
measure) the knee should be strapped with a stretch bandage, or an elastic
half-stocking when a return to sport takes place.

Even after full movement has been restored, either by operative procedures or conservative treatment, and the athlete discharged from medical care, it may take a further two or three weeks before strenuous exercise
should be undertaken. During this period, home treatment by the
sportsman himself is important. The aim is to avoid a recurring injury or
weakness which could happen if the damaged structures were not
returned to full and complete stability. The home treatment exercises
should be continued even after the return to sport to ensure that the
muscles and ligaments are kept at their peak condition.

In order to test that the knee has full extension and full flexion, sit back
on the heels. This should be easy and painless. If it is, do a further test.
While sitting back on the heels put hands on the floor, fingers pointing
away from the body and lean back with a straight back, head dropping
backwards. The main thing, before returning to full activity, is to get full
power in the medial quadriceps muscle down the inner side of the thighs.

Knee Exercise 1

Sit upright on a couch with the legs supported and straight out in front of you, knees relaxed. Tighten the thigh muscle by pressing the knee down on the couch. Exercise both legs though only one has been injured. Do this six times.

Knee Exercise 2

With the injured knee braced, raise the leg upwards then swing it out and across to the other side, back and then down. Repeat the movement on the other side. Do each leg alternately, six times.

Knee Exercise 3

Sit on the edge of the couch with a cushion under the knees and the legs hanging down. Straighten the injured knee firmly. At the same time bend the other knee, pulling the calf hard against the resistance of the couch. Slowly and deliberately change position so that the knee becomes straight, and *vice versa*. Do this six times.

Knee Exercise 4

Lie flat on the floor on a blanket. Bring the feet up along the floor toward the chest, raise the legs in the air and do a bicycling movement with the legs, gently at first and then more vigorously if no pain is felt. Legs together, knees bent, feet on the floor, straighten legs.

HOME TREATMENT AND EXERCISES FOR THE FEET AND ANKLES

Feet can suffer many direct injuries in a variety of sports. They can be hit by hard balls, mallets, hockey sticks and so on; they can be kicked by a horse and they can receive bruises or breakages from being stepped on by cleated shoes. Toes can be broken by stubbing; stress fractures can occur. Strains of the foot are common in many athletic activities. The metatarsal bones at the base of the toes can be fractured by being heavily stepped on, and fallen arches are common to both metatarsal arch (at the base of the toes) and longitudinal (lengthwise) structures.

Ankle sprains are common to many sports. The ankle may rick over while running. Broken ankles occur in snow skiing but sprained ankles are also common in this sport, especially when falls occur in deep, soft snow. A ruptured tendo-Achilles can also result from a similar fall.

Tennis and hurdling may produce tendo-Achilles injuries as well.

In rugby football a direct blow, or people falling over an extended leg in a pile-up, can cause fracture of the ankle bone. The tendo-Achilles and its component muscles in the calf can be strained, torn or ruptured. Muscles can be torn from the shock strain of jumping flat-footed so that the muscles, not being prepared, tear. This can happen in tennis, golf, cricket, volleyball, netball and similar sports.

Before and after returning to a sport following ankle injury, ankle strapping may be advisable, sometimes wrapped around the foot and ankle in a figure-of-eight. The heel or the arch may need to be raised with a rubber pad fitted into the shoe. If there is any sign of swelling when activity again takes place, contrast baths should be taken and the foot rested from weight-bearing until the swelling has gone down.

A group of exercises have been devised to put the joints through their full range of movement and strengthen all related muscles.

Ankle Exercise 1
Sitting on a couch with the knees straight, feet out in front, circle the feet from the ankle, first clockwise, then anti-clockwise: six times each foot.

Ankle Exercise 2
In the same position, turn the soles inward to face each other, then outward, keeping the knees together. Do this six times.

Ankle Exercise 3
In the same position, bend the feet backwards so that the toes point upward, then down so that they point downwards. Repeat six times.

Ankle Exercise 4
In the same position, turn the toes out and pull them up towards the outer sides of the ankles, feeling the pull as you stretch the inside of the ankles and contract the outside. Do this twelve times, then reverse by turning the toes in and pulling the insides of the feet up towards the insides of the ankles: twelve times again.

Toe Exercise 1
In the same position, feet apart and parallel, knees apart and bent, bring the feet upwards and hold. Grip the balls of the feet with the toes and go on gripping to a count of twelve.

Toe Exercise 2

Rest the forefoot so that the base of the toes is resting against something hard, then bend the toes from the ball of the foot, keeping the toe joints straight. Splay the toes and draw them upward, still keeping the toe joints bent. Do this twelve times.

Toe Exercise 3

Stand upright, feet parallel and a few inches apart, raise straight toes off the ground as far as possible. Hold, then curl them under, balancing on the heel. You may hold on to the back of a chair if necessary. Hold for a slow count of six.

Appendix I: Syndesmology

This is the study of that part of the anatomy which deals with joints and their movements. The junction of one bone with another is called a joint.

There are three main types of permanent joints, and these may be classified as:

1. *Synarthroses or Fibrous*

This type of joint occurs in the sutures of the cranium as well as in the occipito-sphenoid and petro-jugular junctions. It is characterised by no cavity, no movement and continuous and direct union of opposing surfaces.

2. *Secondary Cartilaginous Arthroidal*

This occurs in the mid plain as in the symphysis pubis, between each vertebra and the manubrium sterni. If there is an articular cavity it is usually partial or incomplete and there is only partial movement.

3. *Synovial or Diarthrodal*

This type of joint is capable of movement which is controlled by the retaining ligaments. Synovial membrane is present and ends of the bone are covered by hyaline cartilage. In some joints there is a layer of fibro-cartilage between the bone ends as in the menisci of the knee joints. The seven main types of synovial joint may be classified as follows: ball-and-socket; hinge; condyloid; pivot; ellipsoid; saddle; plane.

Ball-and-socket joints allow free movement in all directions; flexion and extension, abduction and adduction, circumduction and rotation. One of the joint surfaces is spheroidal and fits into a cup of similar proportions and slightly greater dimensions. The distal bone is capable of motion around an indefinite number of axes which have one common centre. It is formed by the reception of a globular head into a cup-like cavity, therefore it is multiaxial. Examples are: hip, shoulder, talo-calcaneo-navicular joints (restricted form).

Condyloid joints are modified ball-and-socket joints which allow flexion and extension, abduction, adduction and circumduction. Axial rotation is

223

possible as an accessory 'joint play' movement. There are two distinct pairs of articular surfaces with their long axes almost parallel, and this restricts the movement to one plane. The two pairs of articular surfaces may be enclosed in the same or in different articular surfaces. The motion of condylar joints in uniaxial but slight movement can occur about a second axis. Examples are: wrist and metacarpo-phalangeal joints.

Saddle joints permit freedom of movement in two planes: flexion and extension and abduction and adduction. Each joint surface is saddle-shaped with one apparently inverted and placed at right angles to the other. The opposing surfaces are reciprocal concavo-convex and the motion of the joint is biaxial with rotation in these planes, but not independently. Examples are: carpo-metacarpals of thumb and calcaneo-cuboid.

Hinge joints allow movement in one plane only, flexion and extension. One joint surface is drum or pulley-shaped, and the other is usually slightly cupped to conform approximately with the abutting surface and the bones are connected by strong ligaments. The movement of the joint is uniaxial. Examples are: interphalangeal, talocrural and humero-ulnar. The knee is a modified hinge joint.

Pivot joints are formed by a pivot turning within a ring, or a ring turning on a pivot formed partly of bone and ligament, and allow only one movement – that of rotation. Therefore pivot joints are uniaxial in motion. Examples are: dens-atlas, median atlanto-axial, proximal radio-ulnar and distal radio-ulnar.

Plane joints are formed by the opposition of nearly flat articular surfaces and the gliding movements are restricted by ligaments or osseous processes around the articulation. Gliding is the only movement performed by plane joints. Examples are: acromio-clavicular, lateral atlantoaxial, articular process of vertebrae (facet joints) costo-vertebral, intercarpal, metacarpal, sacroiliac (irregular), tibio-fibular, cuneo-navicular, inter-cuneiform, cuneo-cuboid, tarso-metatarsal, and intermetatarsal.

Ellipsoid joints are those in which an oval convex articular surface is received into an elliptical concavity so as to permit flexion, extension, abduction, adduction and circumduction. The motion of ellipsoid joints is biaxial. Examples are: atlantoaxial, radiocarpal, metacarpophalangeal and metatarsophalangeal joints.

The bones forming the joints are sealed together by a fibrous capsule which is strengthened at certain points, particularly at both the sides, in the front and at the back, by strengthening ligaments. Inside the fibrous capsule is the synovial membrane which secretes the synovial fluid, thus allowing the bones to move smoothly, one on the other. Outside the joint capsule there are many soft tissues, all of which play their part in normal joint function. The muscles are so arranged as to make it possible for the joint to move in all directions it accomplishes. The skeletal muscles are made up of red and white fibres which move the joints in their appropriate directions. It is considered by some that the red fibres are concerned with the static fixing action of the muscles, so that the joints are firmly fixed when they are moved by the white fibres, giving joint stability. It is possible in Active Alerted Posture that the fixing action of the muscles is carried out by the strengthening of the red fibres.

The opposing surfaces of the bone are covered by hyaline cartilage, and it is this cartilage which shows the first changes as an epichondritis in osteoarthritis. In certain joints, such as the knee, the sterno-clavicular joint and the temporomandibular joint, there is an interposed fibro-cartilage as intra-articular structures.

Synovial fluid, a viscous fluid enriched by polysaccharides including hyaluric acid, is derived by dialysis from plasma. Its manufacture is affected by abnormal processes such as occur in injury or any form of inflammatory reaction. Synovial fluid lubricates the joints.

Appendix II: The Skeleton

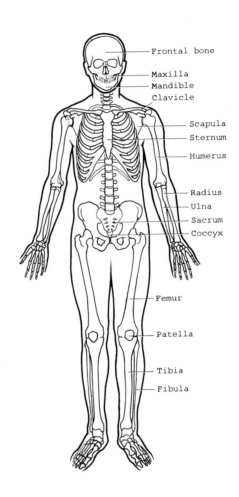

- Frontal bone
- Maxilla
- Mandible
- Clavicle
- Scapula
- Sternum
- Humerus
- Radius
- Ulna
- Sacrum
- Coccyx
- Femur
- Patella
- Tibia
- Fibula

References and Further Reading

American Academy of Orthopaedic Surgery, *Joint Motion Method of Measuring and Recording* (Cassells and Livingstone, Edinburgh, 1966)

Apley, A. G., *A System of Orthopaedics and Fractures* (Butterworth, London, fourth edition 1973)

Berland, T., and Addison, R. G., *Living with your Bad Back* (Pelham Books, London, 1973)

Central Council of Physical Education, *Planning for Sport* (published for the Sports Council, London, 1968)

Committee on Injuries of the American Council of Orthopaedic Surgeons, *Emergency Care and Transportation of the Sick and Injured* (Banter, Menasha, Wisconsin, USA, 1971)

Corrigan and Morton, *Get Fit the Champion Way* (Souvenir Press, London, 1968)

Crawford Adams, J., *Outline of Fractures* (Livingstone, Edinburgh, 1972)

Crawford Adams, J., *Outline of Orthopaedics* (Livingstone, Edinburgh, sixth edition 1977)

De Lorne, T. L., 'Restoration of Muscle Power by Heavy Resistance Exercises', *Journal of Bone and Joint Surgery*, vol. 27B, p. 645 (1968)

Freiberger, R. H., and Halpern, M., *Orthopaedic Radiology in Modern Trends in Orthopaedics* (Butterworth, London, 1967)

Giannestras, N. J., *Foot Disorders: Medical and Surgical Management* (Lea and Feriger, New York, second edition 1973)

Helfet, A., *Disorders of the Knee* (Lippincott, Philadelphia, 1974)

Jesse, John, *Hidden Causes of Injury, Prevention and Correction for Running Athletes and Joggers* (Athletic Press, Pasadena, California, 1977)

Kraus, H., *Backache, Stress and Tension* (Simon & Schuster, New York, 1965)

London, P. S., *A Practical Guide to the Care of the Injured* (Livingstone, Edinburgh, 1967)

Mercer, W., and Duthie, R. B., *Orthopaedic Surgery* (Edward Arnold, London, 1964)

McGregor, A. L., *Anatomy* (Wright, Bristol, 1957)

O'Donaghue, D. H., *Treatment of Injuries in Athletes* (W. B. Saunders, Philadelphia, second edition 1970)

Perkins, G., *Orthopaedics* (London University Athlone Press, 1962)

Seddon, H. J., 'Classical Nerve Injuries', *British Medical Journal*, 2, p. 237 (1942)

Smillie, I. S., *Injuries of the Knee Joint* (Livingstone, Edinburgh, 1970)

Tucker, W. E., and Armstrong, J. R., *Injury in Sport* (Staples Press, London, 1964; now out of print but obtainable in most libraries)

Tucker, W. E., *Posture and Home Treatment in Injury, Rheumatism and Osteoarthritis* (Livingstone, Edinburgh, 1973)

Tucker, W. E., 'Athletic and Industrial Muscle and Joint Injuries' in Robb, C., and Smith, R., *Clinical Surgery* (Butterworth, London, 1964)

Warwick, R., and Williams, P. L. (editors), *Gray's Anatomy* (Livingstone, Edinburgh, thirty-fifth edition 1973)

Williams, J. G. P., and Speryn, P. N., *Sports Medicine* (Edward Arnold, London, second edition 1976)

Wynn Parry, C. B., 'Electrodiagnosis', *Journal of Bone and Joint Surgery*, vol. 43B, p. 222 (1961)

Index

Abdominal strains from rowing, 86
Abduction eversion, 143, 145
Abrasions, 63, 68, 71–2
Accident(s), factors influencing, 98
  proneness to, cure for, 98
Acromiectomy for shoulder injury, 200
Acromio-clavicular joint, dislocation, 203
  graft for, 203
  subluxation of, 202–3
Activator muscle action, 22, 24
Active Alerted Posture, 15, 16, 17, 18, 145, 146
  for back injury, 173, 175
  in rehabilitation, 207
Active Therapeutic (AT) Approach to recovery, 92–206
Adduction inversion, 143
Adductors, injuries, exercise for, 32
Air embolism from scuba diving, 82
Air splints, 44
Alexander method of exercise, 29
American Academy of Orthopaedic Surgeons, tips from, 49–51
American football injuries in 66, 67
Amino acids, 26
Anatomy and pathology of athletic injuries, 93–100
Angling, injuries from, 87
Ankle(s), bath exercises for, 209
  dislocation of, 40
  and foot, anatomy of, 141–2
  home treatment and exercises for, 220–2
  injuries to, 89, 143–6
  sprained, 54, 220
  unstable, exercise for, 145
Annoxia from scuba diving, 81
Anterior cruciate ligament injury, 154
Anterior tibial compartment syndrome, 149–50
Antiphlogistine poultice, 113
Anti-tetanus injections for game shooters, 73
Arms and elbows, home treatment for, 213

Arnica for bruising, 62
Arterial circulation function, 20
Arthrography, 101
  and correct diagnosis, 152–3
Arthropad for knee injury, 59
Arthroscopy, 102, 153
Articular cartilage, 96
Artificial grass, injuries from, 70
Artificial respiration, 75–6
  machine for, danger of incorrect usage, 81
Asphyxia from diving accident, 76
Aspiration of haematoma, 121
Association football injuries, 63–7
Association for the Study of Problems of Internal Fixation (AO), 133
Athlete(s), body movement and, 23
  calory intake, 26
  diet of, 28
  fitness of, 15
  mental preparation, 30–1
  protein for, 26
  and weight lifting, 29
Athlete's foot from swimming pools, 78
Athletic injuries, anatomy and pathology, 63–100
Athletics, first-aid in, 52–5
Atlanto-axial joint, 20
Australian football injuries, 63–7
Australian stretcher for spinal injuries, 57
Avalanches, precautions and dangers, 88
Axonotmesis, 128

Back, exercises for, 217
  injury treatment, 173
  and neck injuries, 169
  supports, 172
Badminton injuries, 70–2
Baer's tender point in sacroiliac injury diagnosis, 167
Ball-and-socket joints, 20, 223
Baseball finger, 59
Baseball, injuries, 57–60
  posture in, 23–4

Basketball injuries, 57–60
Bath exercises, 208–9
Bed rest inactivity and circulation, 21
Bends from scuba diving, 80–1
Blast injury from diving, 77
Bleeding, signs, symptoms and treatment, 50
Blisters, foot, 25
  from rowing and sculling, 86
Blood, analysis, 102
  clotting in legs from cycling, 68
  collection in haematoma, absorption of, 120
  vessels, injury to, 36–7
Blue unconsciousness, 51
Boating injuries, 85–6
Bob-sledding injuries, 89–90
Body fluid, 21
Body mechanics, 15
Body movement, mechanics of, 18
Body muscle function, 22
Bones, 18, 19
  broken, vitamin C for, 28
  direct injury to, 122
  dislocation and pressure on nerve, 40
  grafting in low back pain, 175
  structural defect and low back pain, 175
  vitamins for, 27
  See also Fractures
Bourbon sling, 44
Boxers, concussion of, enforced rest for, 178
Boxing injuries, 60–2, 181
Brachial neuritis treatment, 112
Brain and movement, 22–3
Breathing exercises for rib cage and thoracic wall injury, 179
  value of, 29
Bruised heel, 53
Bruises, 56, 63, 68, 71
Burns, from bob-sledding, 90
  degrees of, 69
  first-aid for, 69
  from motor racing, 69

229

Bursae, effect of injury or gout on, 126, 127
ileo-psoas, 127
impeding recovery, 96
prepatellar, 126–7
semimembranosus, 127
sub-acromial 127
treatment, 127
tuber ischii, 127
Bursitis, an angling injury, 87
associated with tennis elbow, 189
Buttocks, injuries of, 57

Calcium deposits in shoulder, 199
Calf muscle, injury, exercise for, 32, 33
tears and strains, 60, 65, 71
Canadian Air Force method of exercise, 29
Canoeing injuries, 86–7
Capitellum, osteochondroma of, 185–6
Capsule, joint, injury to, 20, 37, 40
Capsulitis in shoulder injury, 195, 200
manipulation for, 198
Carbohydrates, in diet, 28
origin and function, 26, 27
Cardio-pulmonary resuscitation, tips for, 49
Carpal joints, contusions and sprains, 204
Carpo-metacarpal joints, 20
injuries to, AT approach, 180–3
Carpal scaphoid, fixation of, 139
fracture treatment, 181
operation for reduction of, 182
Cartilage, articular, treatment, 125
Cartilaginous rings of vertebral body, 169
Cauliflower ears, 62, 63
Central nervous system, disease of, and unconsciousness, 35
Cerebral cortex, injury to, 35
Cervical spine, fracture, paralysis in 42
fracture-dislocation, 175
and osteoarthritis, 171
unstable fracture and grafting, 175–6
Cervical torticollis, effect of, 171
Cervical vertebral joints, sprains of, 202
Charleyhorse, localised intramuscular tear, 59, 217

Check brace for clavicle injury, 200
Cheek bruising from gun recoil, 73
Chondro-epiphysitis of growing epiphyses, 191
Chondromalacia, 152, 158, 159, 204
Chondrotin sulphuric acid in weight-bearing bones, 96
Circuit training, 30
Circulation, of body fluid, 21
estimation of in injured part, 97
pool exercises for, 210
Clavicle, dislocation and fractures of, 56, 65, 212
operation for, 201, 202, 203
rings for immobilisation, 202
strapping for, 200, 201, 202
Climate, disabilities caused by, 54–55
Clothing, suitable, in training, 25
Coccyx, 19
Cold therapy, 107, 112
Cold weather, effects of, 55
Collarbone, see Clavicle
Collar and cuff sling, 44
Comminuted fracture, 130
Common sports injuries, 117–30
Comparative injuries in various sports, 48
Compression, method of application, 102
Concussion, 177–8
bleeding with, 178
causes of, 66
first-aid for, 58
from motor racing, 69–70
rest for, 70
resting of sportsman after, 66
signs, symptoms and treatment, 50
Condyloid joint, 20, 223
Contact injuries, protective clothing for, 24, 66
Contrast baths, 148
in rehabilitation, 207–8
for strains and sprains, 75
Contused tissues, necrotic, removal of, 125
Contusions, 36, 37, 52, 56, 125
from football, 63
from ice hockey, 90
treatment, 56
Contusion sprain of foot, 147
Convulsions, signs, symptoms and treatment, 51
in oxygen poisoning, 81

Coral, injuries from, 80
Cradle arm sling, 44
Cramp, muscle, 25
Cricket, injuries, 57–60, 168
posture in, 23
Cross-country running injurie 52–5
Cuts and bruises, 52, 53, 63
Cycle racing injuries, 67–8

Decompression sickness from scub diving, 80
De Cussie method in America football treatment, 67
Degenerative changes and low bac pain, 174
De Goes, humeral meniscus of, 19
Dehydration and cramp, 25
Depressed fracture of skull, 35
Diabetic coma, signs, symptom and treatment, 35, 50
Diathesis, septic, toxic and gout 204
Diet, balanced, 28. See also Nutr tion
Direct blows, first-aid for, 58
Direct injury, 58
to bone, 122
haematoma with, 119
to joints, 122
recovery time, 118–23
Disc, intervertebral, see Interve tebral disc
Discus throwers, weight lifting fo 29
Discus throwing injuries, 52–5
Dislocations, 39, 40, 64–5
complications of, 40
partial, 39
and subluxations, 212
Diving injuries, 77–8
training for, 83
Dorsal vertebrae, upper, compre sion of, 176
and fibrositic changes, 171
paralysis in, 42
Drowning, first-aid for, 75–6
Drug addiction in diagnosis unconsciousness, 35
Drunkenness, signs, symptoms ar treatment, 50

Ear, injury in rugby, 64
drum rupture from scuba divin 82

Effusions, of joints, aspiration of, 122
synovial, 125
traumatic, removal of, 186
Elbow(s) boxing injuries to, 61–2
bursa on, 127
dislocation of, 40, 41, 65
home treatment for, 213–14
injuries, 186–7
joint, anatomy of, 184–5
injuries to, 185–6
strains, 54
factors for preventing, 190
Electric shock, 51
Electromyographic tests in nerve injuries, 128
Elevation in injury treatment, 102
Ellipsoid joint, 224
Emphysema, subcutaneous, 81
Entrapment, neuritis of dorsal interosseous nerve, 189
syndrome, 129–30
Environment and injured structures, 97
Epilepsy, signs, symptoms and treatment, 50
Epileptic fit, first-aid for, 34, 35
Equestrian sports, injuries, 55–7, 217
Eventing, injuries in, 55
Examination, diagnosis and preliminary treatment, 101–5
Exercises in injury treatment, 106
for back injury, 173
in bath, 208
bicycle, 156
careful grading in recovery, 93
for haematoma absorption, 119
lower extremity, 139, 141
in training, 29, 32–3
Eye injuries, 61, 64, 72, 82
Eyelids, lacerated, first-aid for, 61

Fainting, signs, symptoms and treatment, 50
Faradic stimulation of muscles, 102, 135, 140
Faradic treatment in rehabilitation, 207
See also Faradism
Faradism, 103, 104, 107, 114–15
in fracture treatment, 138
See also Faradic stimulation, treatment
Fartlek, or speed play, 29

Fat(s) in diet, 28
and oils, function of, 26, 27
Fatty pads, enlargement, 159
Fatigue, and scuba diving, 83
and stress fractures, 24, 131, 136–8
AT approach to, 136
Feet and ankles, bath exercises for, 209
home treatment and exercises for, 220–2
painful from ice hockey, 91
pool exercise for, 210
and shins, soreness of, 53
Femoral condyles, osteochondritis of, 159–60
Femoral fractures, Swiss treatment of, 137
Femur fracture, internal fixation of, 139
Fencing injuries, 62–3
Fibrositis, 94
Fibrous bands, pressure from, 98
thickening, composition of, 99–100
Fibula, fracture of, 43, 52, 65
Field sports, injuries in, 57–60
Fighting sports injuries, 60–3
Finger, dislocation of, 40, 65
fractures, 65
from gun recoil, 74
injuries, 59, 63, 77, 85, 87, 180–3
complication of, 214
home treatment and exercise, 214–16
Fire coral, dermatitis from, 80
First-aid, 34
in specific sports, 52–91
See also specific sports throughout index
First-aid kit, composition of, 48
Fish as protein, 26
Fish hook, removal of, 87
Fitness, and health, 15
and mechanics of movement, 18
exercises, 32–3
Fixation of transverse fractures, 139. See also Internal fixation
Fixed joints, 20
Flat racing injuries, 55, 56
Flexor-pronator strain, 190–1
Food, categories of, 26
and muscle tissue, 20
Foot, blisters, 25
injuries to, 70, 78, 147–8

posture, attention to, 18, 149
strains from golfing, 75
Football, American, protective clothing for, 24
injuries, 35, 63–7, 168, 196, 217
strains in, 38
Footballer's ankle, 146
Forearm injuries, 184
Fractures, 36, 41, 42, 62–3, 65, 68, 87, 89
closed, 131
comminuted, 122, 130
compound, 41, 65, 131
depressed dangers of, 35
fatigue or stress, 24, 131, 136–8, 139
functional activity, 132
haematoma with, 122
hand and fingers, 63, 180–3
immobilisation of, 132, 133
impacted, 143–5
internal fixation of, 133, 136, 139–40
lower extremity, 138
neck and spine, 41
reduction, 132, 137
simple, 40, 131
of skull and unconsciousness, 34–5
splints for, 43–4, 65
transverse, 139–40
of vertebrae, 175–6
Friar's balsam for skin hardening, 86
Frozen shoulder, 197
Fructose, 28
Fungus infection from swimming pools, 78

Gaelic football injuries, 63–7
Game shooting injuries, 72
Garters, tight, and muscle cramp, 25
Gastrocnemius muscle injury, 148
Gauvain brace for spinal injury, 172, 176
Genu recurvatum, 159
Ginglymus composite joint, 184
Gluteal bursa, 127
Golf, injuries, 74–5, 183, 190
strain in, 38
See also Golfer's elbow
Golfer's elbow, 57, 74, 187, 190–1
Gout, 204, 205
diathesis, 169, 190

Gravity, effect on posture, 16, 18
Groin, exercises for, 32
Gun headache, 73
Gun-shot wounds, 72–3

Hand injuries, 59, 61, 180–3
  complications, 214
  fracture of, 40
  home treatment for, 214–16
Haemarthrosis, 37, 57
  from torn synovial membrane,
    125
Haematoma, 37, 60, 164
  affecting recovery, 98
  complications and dangers of
    unabsorbed, 119–20
  effect of undispersed, 99
  with fracture, 122
  swelling, removal of, 103
  treatment for, 120–1
Haemosiderin, 119
Hamstring injury, 163–4, 217
  exercise for, 32
Head and neck injuries, 77, 90
Heart attack in diagnosis of uncon-
    sciousness, 35
  and circulation, vitamins for, 27
Heat, cramps, 55
  exhaustion, 50, 55
  pads, 112, 113
  stroke, signs, symptoms and
    treatment, 25, 50, 55
  therapy, 112
Helfet knee support, 160
Helmets, injuries caused by, 66
Hexcelite splints, 44
Hicks' plates, 184
High jump injuries, 52–5
Hilton's axiom, 93
Hinge joint, 20, 224
Hip(s), bath exercises for, 208, 209
  dislocation and subluxation
    treatment, 40, 166–7
  exercises for, 32
  injuries to, 57
  joint, 20, 165
    ileo-psoas bursa of, 127
    injuries to, 166
  and thighs, home treatment for,
    217–19
  'tight', and tears of rectus femoris,
    162–3
  and hamstring injury, 163
Hockey injuries, 57–60
Home treatment, 207

efficiency essential, 205, 206
  and exercises, 125, 212–22
  for arms and elbows, 213–14
  for fingers, hands and wrists,
    214–16
  for feet and ankles, 220–2
  for hips and thighs, 217–19
  for the knee, 215–20
  joints and sprains, 125
  neck exercises, 210–11
  by patient, 106
  for spine and discs, 216–17
Hospitalisation of sportsmen, 105
Hot baths and rubbing down in
    training, 31
Housemaid's knee, 127
Humerus fracture, internal fixation
    of, 139
Hunting injuries, 55
Hurdling injuries, 55, 221
Hurling injuries, 57–60
Hydrocortisone, anti-flammatory
    action of, 115
  contra-indications to, 116, 149,
    153

Ice, Compression and Elevation
    (ICE) treatment, 75, 102,
    164
  application of, 102
ICE first-aid for strains and sprains,
    75, 118
Ice hockey injuries, 90–1, 218
Ice packs, for bruises, strains and
    contusions, 37, 52, 56, 57,
    58, 59, 60, 67, 112
  for hand injuries, 61
Ileo-psoas, bursa of hip joint, 127
  muscle, short, congenital abnor-
    mality of, 204
Immobilisation of fractures, 43–4,
    65, 132, 133
Impact injuries in fencing, 63
Indirect injury, joints, strains and
    sprains, 125
  muscles and tendons, 123
  recovery time, 123–30
Infection(s), prevention of, 37
  from swimming pools, 78
  and toxic conditions affecting
    healing, 98
Infra-red radiation, 112
Initurf, injuries from, 70
Injection, technique, 107
  therapy, reasons for, 115

Injuries, avoidance and prevention,
    24–5
  common, 34–51
  common sports, 117–30
  comparative, in various sports,
    48
  factors causing, analysed for cor-
    rection, 93, 97, 101
  history of, 101
  retraining after, 15
  soft tissue, 36–7, 117, 137
  unconsciousness, 34–6, 49, 50, 51
  See also specific injuries throughout
    index
Insulin, 51
Intensity duration curves, 128
Intercarpal joint, 20
Interferential current, 105
  therapy, 103, 114
Intermuscular haematoma, 119
Internal fixation of fractures, 133,
    136, 139–40
Internal organs and posture, 18
Interval running in training, 29–30
Intervertebral discs, 169
  home treatment for, 216
  injury in fencing, 62
  involvement causing back pain,
    172
  removal of, 174
Intervertebral joints, strains and
    sprains of facet, 172
Intracranial haemorrhage affecting
    posterior meningeal artery,
    danger from concussion, 178
Intramuscular tear, localised, 59
Intramuscular type of haematoma,
    119, 120
Isometric exercises, 118, 135, 155,
    157, 177
  between treatments, 103
  in fractures, 132, 138
  for joint dislocation, 127
  in rehabilitation, 207
  in training, 29

Jacksonian fits from skull fracture,
    35
J'ai alai, injury from, 72
Jammed finger in basketball, 59
Javelin throwing injuries, 52–5, 191
Jellyfish, injury from, 79
Jogging on the spot exercise, 29
Johanson, Doctor Otto, compara-
    tive injury statistics, 48

Joints, anatomy of, 224–5
  ankle, 141, 142
  direct injury to, 122–3
  dislocation of, reduction and treatment, 127–8
  exercise of in fractures, 132
  hand and fingers, injuries to, 180–3
  injuries to, 37
    aftercare, 204
    danger of immediate strapping, 205
    swelling during treatment, 205
  kinds of, 19–20
  laxity, general, the unstable knee, 160–1
  of Lushka, 171
  manipulation, 206
  strains and sprains, ultrasound therapy for, 94, 114
    aspiration of effusion, 122
    internal derangement, 125
    treatment, 125
  subluxation of, recovery time, 127
  types, 223

Kaolin poultice, 113
Knee(s), cap, bursae on, 126–7
  cartilage, tearing of, 65–6
  and circulation, pool exercise for, 210
  dislocation of, 40
  home treatment and exercises for, 219–20
  injuries, 59, 70, 219
  joint, 150–1
    injuries to and consequent pathological conditon, 151–2
    unstable, causes and treatment, 160–1
Knuckles and hands, injuries from boxing, 61
Küntscher nail for fractures, 137, 140, 183
  and Phemister grafting, 140

Lacrosse injuries, 57–60
Lateral (talo-fibular) ligament, injuries to, 143–4
  pivot shift, 161
Laughton Scott solution in injection therapy, 116
Leg cartilages, injuries to, 66
LIFE (Lumbar, Isometric, Flexion, Exercise), 173, 216

Ligament(s), 20
  damage to in dislocation, 40
  in sprains, 39
  in strains, 38
Liver, 27
Low back pain, causes, 174
Lower back, bath exercises for, 208, 209
Lower extremity, 140–2
  fractures, 138–9
  spine, bath exercises for, 208
Lumbago, 170
L.5/S.1 facet joint, muscle spasm from, 167
Lumbar region, manipulation, 173
  spinal fracture paralysis, 42
  vertebrae, 19
Lung injury from scuba diving, 82
Luskha, joints of, 171
Lymphatic circulation, 20

McBurney's point, 167
McKee brace for spinal injury, 172
Manipulation, under general anaesthetic, 112
  and mobilisation techniques, 107, 108
  of shortened muscles, 110–12
  treatment, rule of, 105, 111–12
March fractures, 136
Mechanical sports, injuries from, 67–70
Medial collateral ligament injury, 154, 157
Medial meniscus, damage to, 154, 157, 158
Medial tibio-femoral compartment, derangement of, 162
Medilintex poultice, 113
Meniscus injuries, 154, 157, 158
Mennell's test for sacroiliac joint injury, 167
Mensendieck exercise system, 29
Mental preparation for sport, 30
Metacarpal fracture, fixation of, 139
Metacarpo-phalangeal joints, injury to, AT approach, 180–3
Metatarsal bones, fatigue fracture, 43
  fracture of, AT approach, 52, 147
  transverse fracture, 181
Micro-wave therapy, 103, 105, 112, 113
Milk in diet, 27
Minerva plastic collar, 175

Molten wax for heat treatment, 112, 113
Motor cycle racing injuries, 68
Motor racing injuries, 68–70
Mouth-to-mouth resuscitation, 76
Mouth-to-nose resuscitation, 76
Movement(s), muscle and, 22
  incorrect execution and injury, 94
Muscle(s), activator, 22, 24
  antagonist, 22, 100
  cramps, 25
  fibrotic, 119
  injury to, 36
  nerves in, 22
  prime fixors, 22
  pulled, causes, 25
  and sciatica, 173
  spasm in, 173
  sprain, 39
  stimulation in fracture treatment, 135
  strain, 38, 62, 86
    spinal, 172
  synergist, 22, 24
  tearing, 65, 95
  tissue, needs of, 20
  wasting, 99
Myositis ossificans, 119, 121, 162, 186

Narcosis from scuba diving, 81
Neck, injuries in football, 66
  or spine fractures, 41–2
Nerve(s), affected by entrapment syndrome, 129
  conduction, tests for, 128
  injuries, 128
    recovery time, 128
    surgery for, 128
  involvement in injury, 99
  motor and sensory, 22
  pressure in bone dislocation, 40
Neurapraxia, 128, 129, 199
Neuromuscular mechanism, stimulation of responses, 116
Neurotmesis, 128
Newman's grades of low back pain, 174
Nitrogen poisoning from scuba diving, 81
Nosebleed, 60, 66
Nucleus pulposus of vertebral disc, 109
Nutrition, 15, 26–9
  calories, 26

Nutrition—*contd.*
  carbohydrates, 26, 27
  correct, 25, 26
  protein, 26
  vitamins, 27, 28
  See also Food

O'Donoghue's triad, 154
Odontoid process of axis, fracture
    of, 175
Oedema, cause of, 21
Olecranon, bursa, 127, 186
  fracture, nailing of, 184
  stress or fatigue fracture of, 186,
    191
Open soft tissue wound, 37
Operation, delayed, 104
  early, when necessary, 104
Os calcis, removal of, 148
Osgood's bursa of elbow, 186, 188
Osteoarthritic changes, following
      injury of cervical spine, 171
  in fracture treatment, 138
Osteoarthritis, 95, 162
  of acromio-clavicular joint, 203
  from disc degeneration, 173
  of injured hip, 166–7
  in older sportsmen, 174
  of spine, 73
  of wrist, 183
Osteoarthrosis, 95
Osteochondral erosion, 162
Osteochondral fibrillation, 160
Osteochondritis, 158, 183, 204
  of the femoral condyles, 159
Otitis media from water skiing, 84
Overweight, correction of, 29
Oxygen poisoning in scuba diving,
    81

Paralysis in spinal fracture, 42
Pars interarticularis, fatigue frac-
      ture, 174
  fixation of, 175
Patella, dislocation of, 219
  movement, 151
Pathological findings of injury,
    102
Pelota (jai alai), injury from, 72
Pelvis, 165
  bath exercise for, 208, 209
Penetration injuries in fencing, 62–3
Periosteum, function of, 19
Periostitis associated with tennis
    elbow, 189

Perkins' method of fracture treat-
      ment, 137
Phemister bone slivers, 137, 139
Physiotherapist, treatment by,
    105–6
Physiotherapy, 107
  for joint sprains and strains, 125
Pivot joint, 20, 224
Plane joint, 20, 224
Plaster cast for injury support, 102
Pleurisy, traumatic, from rib injury,
      AT approach to, 180
Poisons, signs, symptoms and
      treatment, 51
Polo injuries, 55, 56–7
Polychloride surfaces, injury from,
    70
Polyvinyl surfaces, injuries from,
    70
Portuguese men o' war, injuries
      from, 79
Posture, 23
  Active Alerted, 15, 16
  and fatigue and stress fractures,
    136
  and foot troubles, 18
  gravity and, 16
  Inactive Slumping, 15
  internal organs and, 18
  lungs, expansion of, 18
  mechanics and body movement,
    18
  poor, effects of, 94
    and degenerative changes, 171
  and spinal injury, 172
Poultices for heat treatment, 112,
    113
Pregnancy and sacroiliac strain, 167
Prepatellar bursa (housemaid's
      knee), 127
Prolapsed disc, 174
Proprioceptive neuromuscular
      facilitation exercise (PNF),
      107, 116
Protective clothing, 24
Protein in diet, 28
  function of, 26
Psychological fitness for sport, 30
Psychosomatic factors in athletics,
    98
Pyramidalis, strain from, 168

Quadriceps injury, exercise for, 32

Racquet sports, 70–2

Radial head, injuries to 185–6
Radius, fibrillation of head of, 189
  fracture of, 40, 41, 65
  internal fixation of, 139
  plating of, 184
Recoil injuries in game shooting,
    73
Recovery, fundamental factors
      affecting, 98–100
  time, 92, 106, 118–30
Rectus abdominis, strain of, 168
Rectus femoris, exercises for, 32
Red unconsciousness, 50
Red, white and blue unconscious-
      ness, 50, 51
Rehabilitation before retraining,
    207–22
Resuscitation methods, 75–6
Retraining after injury, rehabilita-
      tion of, 207–22
Rhythmic stabilisation, 117
Rib cage, injuries to, 178–80
Ribs, bruising and contusion of and
      haematoma, 62, 180
Rower's cramp 86
Rowing, hazards and injuries, 85–6
Rugby injuries, 63–7, 221
Rupture of medial collateral liga-
      ment, 157
Running injuries, 52–5
Rush nail in fracture treatment, 183

Sacroiliac joints, strain or subluxa-
      tion, 167–8
Sacrum, 19
Saddle joints, 20, 224
Salt, lack of, and cramp, 25, 55
  tablets, use of, 55
Scaphoid bone, fracture of, 65
  non-union of, 182–3
  plaster cast for, 181–2
  removal of 181–3, 183–4
  treatment, 181
Sciatica, 171, 175
  and muscle spasm, 173
  of segmental distribution, 173
Scraped skin (abrasions), 57, 58
Scuba diving, contra-indications to,
    83
  injuries, 80
Sculling hazards and injuries, 85–6
Sea fishing injuries, 87
Sea salt in rehabilitation, 208
Sea urchins, danger of, 79
Sea wasp, injury from, 79

Secondary cartilaginous arthroidal joint, 223
Secondary superficial dilatation, 112
Self-manipulation, 211
Self-physiotherapy, 208
Semilunar bone, dislocation of, 182
  replacement of, 182
Semimembranosus, 164
  bursa, 127
Semitendinosus, 164
Sepsis, absorption of, 104
Shin injuries, 59
Shin soreness in fracture of tibia, 136
Shock from burns, 69
  signs, symptoms and treatment, 50
Short-wave diathermy, 103, 105, 112, 113
Shot-putters, injury to, 52–5
Shoulder, dislocation of, 39, 40, 41, 65
  frozen, 197
  girdle, 18
    bath exercise for, 208, 212
  injuries, 62, 74, 85, 87, 193–5
  joint, correct movement of, 191–3, 194
  dislocations, 195–6, 197, 200
  effusion of, 195
  fracture of, 195
  manipulation, 198
  sprain and strain of, 197, 202, 204
  support for, 197
  sprains, 54, 204
  sub-acute and chronic strains and capsulitis, 197, 198
Show jumping, injuries from, 55, 201
Silastic replacement for semilunar bone, 182
Sinus injury from scuba diving, 82
Skeletal framework, function in posture, 18–19
  six levels of, 18–19
Skeleton, 226
Skiing, hazards and injuries, 40, 88–9
Skipping exercises in training, 29
Skull fracture, 41
  signs, symptoms and treatment, 50
Slings, 44
Slocombe repair operation, 161

Slow reversal method in muscle contraction, 117
Snorkeling injuries, 80
Soccer, exercise for, 32
  head injuries in, 35
Soft tissues, bruising, 36
  injuries, 36–7, 148
    closed or simple, 36–7
    defined, 36
    first-aid for, 37
Soleus muscle injury, 148
Sprays for cold therapy, 112
Special events, preparation for, 31
Specific skills, preparation for, 31
Spinal column, 18, 19
  cord, damage to in spine fracture, 42
  fractures, 56
    operations in, 176
    paralysis in, 42, 176, 216
    transportation for, 42
  fusion, when made, 174, 176
  injuries combined with degenerative changes in the disc and spinal joints, 172
    operative treatment, 173
    stretcher for, 57
  nerves, 171
  segment, anatomy of, 169–70
  See also Spine
Spine, fracture of, 41–2
  injury, manipulation for, 173
  pool exercise for, 209–10
Spiral fractures, 181
Splints, fracture, use of, 43–4
  improvised, 43
Split spinal plaster jacket, 176
Spontaneous pneumothorax from scuba diving, 82
Spondylolisthesis, 172
  grades of, 174
Spondylosis, 172, 173, 174
Sports medical facilities, 205
Sprains, 39, 64, 68, 74, 77, 187
  ankle, AT approach to, 143, 144–5
  knee, aspiration of fluid, 153–4
Squash injuries, 70–2
Squeeze injuries from scuba diving, 82
Starches in diet, 27
Steeplechase injuries, 55, 177, 182, 212
Stiffness, beginner's, from water skiing, 84

treatment, 31
Stitch, causes, 25
Strains, 38, 187
  from football, 64
  from golf, 74
  of medial collateral ligament, 157
  from motor cycle racing, 68
  recovery time, 124
  from swimming, 76
'Strawberries' on baseball players, 57
Stress or fatigue fractures, 24, 42–3, 136, 186
Stretch exercise, 32
Stroke, signs, symptoms and treatment, 35, 50
Sub-acromial bursa, 127, 198, 199
Subcutaneous emphysema from scuba diving, 81
Subluxation of joint, 39, 64–5
SUELMEX treatment, 60
Suffocation, signs, symptoms and treatment, 51
Sugars in diet, 27
Sunstroke, 25, 35, 50
  and scuba diving, 83
Supraspinatus syndrome, 62
Supraspinatus tendon calcification, 198
  strain or tear of, 192, 195
Supreme turf, injuries from, 70
Surfing injuries, 85
Surgical spirit for skin hardening, 86
Surgical treatment, types of injury requiring, 103
Swellings of tissue, in AT approach, 103
Swimmer's shoulder, 77
Swimming, injuries, 77–9
  as rehabilitation exercise, 209
Swiss cereal muesli, 28
Swiss Compression System of fracture treatment, 136, 137, 138, 140
Sylvester method of resuscitation, 75
Symphysis pubis, bone grafting for, 168
  disruption of, 168
  injuries to, 168
  muscle movement in, 168
  postural training for pain in, 168
  urethritis and, 168
Synarthroses or fibrous joints, 223

Syndesmology, 223–5
Synergist muscle action, 22, 24
Synovial or diarthrodial joints, 223
Synovial fluid, 225
  effect of injury on, 97
Synovial tuft, 146
Synovitis, 97, 100
  from injury to bursae, 127

Table tennis injuries, 70–2
T'ai Chi Ch'uan method of exercise, 173
Tailor's bursa, 127
Talus, tilted, in ankle injury, 145, 146
Tarsal joints, contusions and sprains, 204
Teeth, damage to in ice hockey, 90
Tendo-Achilles, 124
  injuries to, 65–6, 148
  pulled, 53–4
  rupture of in skiing, 89, 220–1
  tendonitis, linear incision for, 149
Tendons, AT Approach to, 126
  injuries, 25, 126
  recovery time, 126
  rupture of, 98
  sprains and strains, 38, 39
  tearing of, 65
  treatment, 126
  See also Tenosynovitis
Tennis, injuries, 70–2, 183, 221; see also Tennis elbow
  muscle cramp in, 25
  strain in, 38
Tennis elbow, 57, 70, 71, 74, 186, 213
  causes, 187–90
  exercises for, 189
  operation for, 190
  treatment, 189
  factors for preventing elbow strain, 190
Tenosynovitis, 74, 86, 126, 183, 204
Tenovaginitis, 146
Therapy, various forms of, 106–17
Thigh(s), abrasion of, 58
  home treatment and exercise, 217–19
  injury, 60
  muscle injuries, complications, 162–3
  pool exercise for, 209
  strain or tear, 60

Thoracic wall and rib cage, injuries to, 179–80
  support for, 180
Thrombophlebitis from cycling, 68
Thrower's shoulder, 54
Thumb joint, strain of in polo, 57
Tibia and fibula fracture, internal fixation for, 139
  fatigue fracture of, 43
  fracture of, 65
Tibio-fibular joint, loss of movement in, 150
Tight joint, 204
Tincture of benzoin for skin hardening, 86
Tinel's sign in nerve injury recovery, 128
Tissue, necrosis, 118
  reaction to injury, 115
  tenderness, causes of, 100
Toe(s) exercises, 222
  pain in, 54
Tourniquet, application and precautions, 45
Toxoid injections for game shooters, 73
Traction and activity method for fracture treatment, 137, 140
Trainer assisting physiotherapist, 106
Training, general, 15, 29–30
  exercise, 32–3
  mental preparation, 30
  special events, 31
  specific skills, 31
Transverse fracture of hand, 181
Transverse process of vertebrae, fracture of, 176–7
Transverse spinal cord paralysis, cause of, 176
Traumatic effusion, removal of, 99, 102, 104
  swelling, components preventing recovery, 98–9
  syndromes, phases and stages, 97
Treatment, factors related to, 96–7
'Treat and train' motto, 204
Tuber ischii, 127

Ulna, fracture of, 40, 41, 65
  internal fixation of, 139
  partial removal in tenosynovitis, 183
Ultrasound therapy, 103, 105, 112, 113–14

Unconsciousness in sport, causes and diagnosis, 34–6
  tips from American Academy o Orthopaedic Surgeons, 49
Upper extremity, injuries to 180–203
Urethritis and painful symphysis pubis, 168

Varicose veins from cycling, 67
Varidase for bruising, 62
Vascular disorders from cycle racing, 67
Venous circulation function, 20
Vertebrae, 19
Vertebral body, 169
Vertebral column, fractures in volving, 175–6
Vitamins, A and D, origin and function, 27
  B group complex, 27–8
  C origin and function, 28
Volkmann's ischaemic contracture in elbow injury, 104, 187

Waist and top half of spine, pool exercises for, 209
Waste products, elimination of, 20, 94
Water skiing, clothing for, 84
  hazards of, 84–5
Water polo, hazards and injuries, 85
Water sports, injuries from, 75–87
Wax baths, 102, 105
Weals, treatment for, 63
Weight lifting, for athletes, 29
  benefit of, 29
White unconsciousness, 50, 51
Winter sports, injuries from, 88–91
Wire ladder splints, 44
Wounds, closed or simple, 36
  healing precautions, 105
  open soft tissue, 37
  toilet in open fractures, 131
Wrist, fracture of, 40
  home treatment and exercises for, 214–15
  injury, 57
  sprains from swimming, 77

X-rays, 101

Yachting injuries, 87
Yeast, 27
Yoga, 29